portion size me

A Kid-Driven Plan to a Healthier Family

Marshall Reid and Alexandra Reid

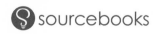
sourcebooks

Published by Sourcebooks, Inc.
P.O. Box 4410, Naperville, Illinois 60567-4410
(630) 961-3900
Fax: (630) 961-2168
www.sourcebooks.com

Library of Congress Cataloging-in-Publication data is on file with the publisher.

Printed and bound in the United States of America.
VP 10 9 8 7 6 5 4 3 2

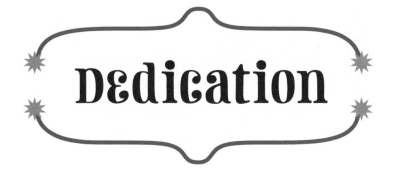

Dedication

I'd like to dedicate this book to kids who have been put in my situation and have been bullied to the point of embarrassment and disbelief in themselves. I have done this to help you stand up and say "no" to being scared and sad from being unhealthy. And to encourage you to stand up and be confident in yourself. It's OK to be happy, you're allowed.

Marshall

Dear Reader: This book is dedicated to you; for you have some desire within you to honor and respect your body; to capture and cultivate a positive sense of self; and to restore or renew a happy, healthy, and fun environment to your kitchens and your homes. And my hope is, much the way Marshall inspired our family, that you will share your experiences and journeys and inspire others to consider the care and upkeep of their human vessels. After all, you can't change without making a change!

Kindly,

Alex Reid

2024

contents

Acknowledgments

Marshall: I could not have done this without my mommy. My mom has been a great inspiration to me. And she has pushed me with the project and writing this book, in a good way. I would like to specifically thank all who have subscribed to the Portion Size Me YouTube channel for their encouragement and the belief they have given me throughout this project. We have gotten comments on our website and other places too. It's those comments, from total strangers, that really inspire me and I want to thank you all for taking the time to leave them.

Alex: It is with sincere and heartfelt gratitude and appreciation that I extend a big "Thank You" to: Marshall, Jordan, Dan, Terri, Jenks, Pilar, Nikki, Leslie, Kim, Sourcebooks, Kelly, Steve, CNN, Nate Berkus, and Jamie Oliver!

Introduction

Meet Marshall

Hi, my name is Marshall Reid. When I was ten, I asked my mom if we could do the opposite of the *Super Size Me* documentary and be healthy for a month. *Super Size Me* is that movie where a guy ate McDonald's for thirty days. I asked to do this because my classmates were making fun of me and I didn't feel good. I couldn't run and keep up. I wasn't fast enough to play tag and ball with kids at recess. And I always pulled on my clothes to keep them from creeping up on my stomach. We ate out a lot and I snacked a lot. I just felt like something had to change because I was getting really unhappy. I was worried that I was always going to feel that way.

I was happy my mom listened, and we sat down together and talked about what we thought "healthy" meant to us. We decided on some things that we thought sounded reasonable to us, like cooking more and reading ingredients. We talked a lot about changing habits and making new ones—good ones for a lifetime. My mom asked me if there were people I wanted to be like. She asked me how I wanted to feel when I was a teenager and when I was an adult. It helped me to picture in my mind how to get to those feelings. My mom, sister, and I talked a lot about physical activity and exercise. My mom asked me what kinds of foods I liked and if I would help her in the kitchen. We decided to call our project Portion Size Me because it was similar to but opposite of that movie, and a part of our problem was that we just ate too much!

We have had lots of fun and many adventures with this project, and we wanted to share them with you. In fact, it's not just a project anymore. It has become our life. It isn't always easy, but I will tell you that it does get easier and easier as you keep going.

This book is a mix of two types of books: a cookbook and the story of my family's journey to healthier living. I don't want to spoil the story, so I'm not saying anything other than it was a success! So come on, let's Portion Size Me!

Meet Marshall's Mom (aka Alex)

Portion Size Me came from the mouth of babes. My babe! And I am so proud of him!

When Marshall suggested the concept, I was excited for a project to do together that would unite us and perhaps even help him build his self-esteem. He is such a rich and colorful young person, and I want him to feel good about sharing his personality and to not feel inhibited because of his self-image or feel sad because of playground meanness. I was very surprised that he identified and spoke out about his needs at only ten years old. The internal strength it must have taken him, and the self-awareness and ability to put it into words, are among the many traits that make him a dynamic and colorful personality. I knew right away this project was going to be very good for all of us.

As we got underway and I began to observe our habits from a new and fresh perspective, it became clear to me that some absences and voids needed to be addressed. In particular, I noticed the absence of proper respect for food and focus on its nutritional value, and the void of good habits and the self-discipline to back up those habits. After just a few conversations with Marshall about how we were going to lay this project out, it occurred to me that I was the one responsible for not empowering Marshall with the healthy connections to food that would follow him into adulthood. I learned from Marshall that he had become an emotional eater and not a fuel-driven eater. That made me worry that, as an adult, he would continue to turn to food for comfort and other emotional needs instead of feeling the simple joyful appreciation of food's ability to keep one's body functioning.

Once Marshall and I agreed on our Portion Size Me goals, I next had to figure out how to incorporate them into our very busy schedules. After all, I believe our schedules were what began to dictate our food choices for convenience's sake. I looked for ways to simplify our schedules and organize my time better, such as writing out a grocery list for a week at a time instead of stopping by the store every other day to pick up a few quick things.

I looked at the kitchen from a historical perspective, and I then considered the modern technologies developed to aid with cooking. I spoke with my neighbor, who already has grown children, and a few friends about how they felt about their kitchens. I don't mean what appliances they had, how their cabinets looked, or whether or not they liked the design of their kitchens, but rather the emotions and feelings their kitchens evoked. Why is it, for example, that whenever you entertain, everyone lingers in the kitchen despite other wide-open spaces with comfy couches and tables? I believe it's because we know that the kitchen is a source of comfort and the place where one builds connections with others.

I searched my memories of childhood and the foundation of my relationship with food. Unlike my husband Dan, who grew up on a farm, I grew up in a small town in Northern California. I saw vineyards and farms and cattle, but I pretty much believed everything was born, raised, and packaged at the local grocery store. It was a safe naïveté because food in our household was always very carefully counted for the sake of calories by the head of household. Fresh fruit and skinless chicken where staples, and I, as a pre-teen, was the primary cook for the house. There wasn't any joy in it; it was a chore. Occasionally, I was provided with the ingredients and picture of a beautiful dish cut from the pages of a fashion or interior design magazine and asked to put it together. That was stressful, as there was a lot of pressure to make the meal correctly. Later, as a young adult in Manhattan attending school and working, cheap became my culinary focus; I lived on pizza by the slice and salad bars. So my relationship with food had a rocky and unstable foundation to begin with. Once I could afford to go out to a wonderful New York City restaurant, I do remember feeling an inner smile as I appreciated the colors, designs, and flavors on my plates. It was during this time that I took advantage of NYC's international flavor and really began to open up my palate to different cultures and their cuisines. My ideas of food began to change as I met many different people and explored new locations to enjoy food. Eating out became a form of entertainment and a social medium, which was also not an entirely healthy relationship with food.

So, that was one of our goals: to return to the kitchen and create real, delicious, and nourishing meals. To step back and refocus the importance of the kitchen and the family's participation in creating fuel for our active vessels. We decided to document the experience via home videos for a couple of reasons. First it was to be "documentary" in style like *Super Size Me*. Second, we had just discovered Skype video calls with Dan in Iraq. This new access to media was a big help to our family during his deployment, but there was a big time change. So we thought if we posted videos, Dan could watch them and then we could all Skype about them at a later time. The third purpose for creating videos was to hold us accountable to our goals. It was an outside source that we had a responsibility to keep up with. Neither Marshall nor I had any idea he would be so good on camera; we had never done anything like it. None of the videos you see are rehearsed or directed, and we have only had a handful of retakes due to excessive giggling or distraction from a friend or dog.

I am so happy to share our experiences with you. I am not embarrassed to share my failures with you either. We promise not to tell you to do this or to do that; we are simply sharing what we have learned and the impact that our adventure has had on us. We also promise not to bombard you with lots of heavy research and statistics. For example, it is up to you to form your own opinion on whether or not milk pasteurization is for you or whether you want to eat all organic foods. We will, however, provide you with a brief definition of certain terms so that you may look into them further if you wish. We are sharing some of our favorite recipes that are uncomplicated and direct, plus some culinary terms and definitions to make cooking fun and enlightening. We're including history and folklore accounts of food to use as tools to spur conversation and association with particular recipes. And of course, Marshall's charm and inspiration follow you through this book.

I hope our family's examination of what has become such a common problem in the United States today, and our solution for becoming healthy become tools and solutions for you and your family. We as a country are on a path to a disease-filled future, robbing us of our hard-earned dollars for the sake of healthcare treatments and costs that could have been prevented. I hope that if you are a child or the parent of a child reading this book, you will relate to the struggles we identified and feel encouraged that you are not alone. You can be strong, regain control, and feel as good as you possibly want to feel!

Meet Marshall's Sister (aka Jordan)

Hi! I'm Jordan. At the beginning of summer, we decided to try to be healthier! My mom has always told me that I need to put on some "fighting weight" because I have always been athletic and on the thinner side of the weight scale. My case is the exact opposite of my brother's. But both cases can be helped by just eating healthier foods! See, I like junk food. A LOT! Candy and chips are my favorite. Many of my friends only drink soda, and it is starting to show on them. I learned during this project that my body wasn't getting the nutrition it needed. Healthier food does make a difference! Just because you're thin doesn't mean you're healthier than overweight people. I have been to farms and grown vegetables and herbs at home. I know how seeds start and grow and how much care farmers put into growing crops. It makes me appreciate what they do and how good the food is for you. These days, I would much rather stroll down the aisles of the farmers' market and take in the colors and smells of the fresh food than walk down the Walmart aisles and grab a bag of something. Wouldn't you?

Meet Marshall and Jordan's Dad (aka Dan)

The way I was raised certainly affected the way I view food. I grew up on a farm in Iowa that provided about 70 percent of the foods we ate. We raised our own livestock for meat and chickens for eggs, and my dad always had a huge garden each summer that pro-vided us with corn, tomatoes, beans, peas, and squash throughout the year. In addition, we traded meats and vegetables with neighbors to add to the table. Every meal focused on meat and potatoes, with a vegetable side.

My childhood activities also influenced the way we ate. TV had only four channels, and while my brother had an Atari video-game system, video games were things that didn't attract me. Instead, I was either reading or outside roaming the farm and fields looking for excitement. This meant that I was active after school and on the weekends. To make sure I had plenty of energy, meals were always large affairs. Breakfast was either cereal or eggs and bacon. Lunch was sandwiches and soup. Dinner was always the biggest meal of the day, with huge portions of meat, potatoes, and side dishes. Salads were uncommon, although we did occasionally have them on the side (never for the main course). We were allowed to eat as much as we wanted and not only encouraged to clean our plates, but required to.

When I left home for college, my views of food changed drastically. Food was only fuel for me. I ate only because I had to, and I did so as cheaply and quickly as possible. The old joke about surviving on Ramen noodles and Kool-Aid was my reality. Instead of taking the time to think about what I put into my body, I adopted the "grab and go" mentality. Meals were a distraction, and I lost the ability to enjoy not only the food, but also the social process of eating and enjoying the time with my friends and family. The foods that I ate changed as well. Gone were the homemade dishes and fresh meats and vegetables. Instead I ate canned anything and frozen everything.

My adult life and career in the military have helped me experience many different aspects of food. I have been fortunate to live in other countries for extended periods of time, allowing me to test and taste the foods of other cultures. In Korea, I saw the blending of minimal meats with really fresh veggies and flavorful, light sauces. In Kenya, I tasted roasted meats with few to no spices, allowing the meat to stand on its own. In Egypt and Iraq, I was treated to traditional meals of rice, chicken, and dates with healthy doses of cumin and curry. All of these cultures presented different flavors and textures. But the biggest impression I got from all of them was that they treated food not only as fuel, but also as a social event. In every one of these countries, we sat down to a meal as an event. Instead of rushing through the meal, we sat and enjoyed the foods and the process of eating them.

Today, the vestiges of my childhood still form my concepts of a meal. Large portions, meat and potatoes, and few light alternatives. As I have gotten older, I have had to realize that the way I eat may not be in concert with the way my body reacts to the foods I put into it. But Marshall has helped me see other options, and I feel the benefits. Fruits, something I never really had much of as a child, are now front and center for breakfast. Salads and light fare for lunch and dinner, with a focus on portion control, have helped me to change my eating habits in a good way, especially as I get older and my metabolism changes.

Portion Size Me Goals

This is not a diet, plan, or program that we created to rigidly follow. This is a lifestyle. It is about putting food in the spotlight, at the forefront of your mind, and viewing it as beautiful, nutrient-rich fuel to energize one's body and soul. We want to be happy and fulfilled—never feeling robbed or restricted. We want to explore and be food adventurers. We can think of ourselves as our own personal chefs, and we can create delicious meals that avoid the extremes that may have derailed us in the past. Even if a situation arises where the best choice cannot be made, a mind-set of moderation still guides us. We just make the next choice the best choice.

With *Portion Size Me*, we want to change our unsuccessful behaviors slowly, and we want to enjoy every moment with our families and with ourselves as we begin to feel positive changes occurring. This is our commonsense approach, and there is no miracle to it—just thoughtful consideration, planning, and patience. For example, Marshall suggested to his elementary school that they create a healthier lunch just once a month, so that there's not too much impact on the school budget. He then suggested that the following year, they serve the new, healthier lunch once a week, and the year after that, twice a week. And so on. That way they can plan and ease into the budget changes. Slow and steady! That is a wonderful example of moderation and avoiding an extreme change that could be viewed as a barrier.

Our new attitude is that food is the tool, the fuel, and the fire that propels your body to function through your day and throughout your life. Our food choices and the quantities we eat have been problems, but food is also part of the solution. We are going to embrace it, harness it, and own it to make us feel better and stronger, and help us look the way we want to. This book shows how we are going to make that emotional and attitudinal shift toward food.

Our Goals

Eat as Many Real Foods as Possible

#1: For us, real food is food that is made from a combination of natural products, or is by itself a single natural product. Real food comes from a once-living source. In addition to eating as much real food as we can, another part of this goal is to try to choose local products whenever possible to support our nearby farmers and our community.

Fresh fruits, vegetables, fish, and meats are obvious choices for "real" products. We are not suggesting that you have to purchase all of your meats from a local farm, although that would be great if you did. Instead we would want to choose, for example, a ham steak and baked beans instead of a hot dog with too many ingredients one cannot pronounce in it on a white bun covered in ketchup.

Read Ingredients

#2: The packaged foods we see in grocery stores are effectively billboards promoting each item: telling us what it is, how much it costs, and why it's better than something else. Many government entities and corporations can shout out at you via that packaged communication. It's visual noise, and it's not necessarily in your best interest! How many times do we ignore or not understand the details in that visual message? We want to purposely understand it and make the conscious choice instead of an unconscious one.

You can spend hours at the grocery store reading everything you purchase and that can be daunting. Who has the time to spend hours at the store? Consider, instead, choosing a handful of products to look at each time you go. You'll start to learn key things to look for (like scientific words you cannot pronounce) and you will start a mental inventory of products you want to add to your cart and those you never want to purchase again. Also, consider picking one word you don't know the meaning of each trip, then coming home and looking it up. This is your life; you have the reins in your hands.

Pause before You Eat

Pausing before you eat allows you to consider what you are about to consume and why. Is this boredom eating? Emotional eating? Exhaustion eating? Laziness? Purposeful pausing allows you to consider, contemplate, and begin enjoying food before you actually have it. Ask yourself if this is the best nutrient-rich food you could choose right now. Is this choice going to allow your body to perform and compete and be able to move onto the next adventure?

This may sometimes be difficult to ask of children, but getting them involved in the food preparation process helps build in natural pauses by way of conversation and sensory exploration, like touching things at the grocery store or helping out in the kitchen.

Get Moving

Exercise. Easier said than done. But physical activity helps to maintain a healthy body. You cannot get anywhere without your body moving. It is your sailing ship, your space vessel, your race car. Your body has something special about it that no one can re-create. It is trainable. Your heart is a muscle that can easily be made stronger to more efficiently pump blood through your system. Your tendons and ligaments can support your structure as you spring into action.

And we can add many small choices in a day to grease the wheels in our joints and keep them moving.

This goal is also to encourage you to get moving in the kitchen and develop your mind-set to view food as fuel.

Help out in the Kitchen

#5: This is a twofold goal. The first is to regularly invite a child to participate with you in the kitchen (or if you are a child reading this book, to ask to participate in the kitchen's daily activities for the education and mindful activity they provide).

Second, a kitchen evokes a story with its history, what it produces, its sense of consistency and routine, and its feeling and comfort. The kitchen is such an interesting place. It has so many jobs. It's the place to sort and organize and yet be comfortable. It's the place of many a smile and good feelings, hugs and wishes for a good day at school or work.

Watch Portion Sizes

#6: We want to remind you that we have become a super-sized, overconsuming nation. Our bodies do not require as much as we are putting in them, and we will not starve to death if we have some reductions in quantity. Marketing themes tell us we are getting a good deal when we order more, and TV cooking shows present culinary delights on large dishes, using the dish as a canvas for their work. But when we purchase beautiful dishes we fill them up instead of viewing them as canvases. Parents dish out servings for kids instead of allowing kids to take their own amounts. Emotional eating, busy schedules, and the idea that food is a reward for a hard day's work all contribute to us just plain eating too much. It's not Thanksgiving every day—just once a year! Our family is a prime example of all of these issues. We regularly have been known to eat dinner until we are uncomfortably full. Yikes.

One of the best things we can do for ourselves is start to monitor and pay attention to the size of the portions we are consuming at each meal. How much do we really need to eat to feel satisfied and full? The answer is often surprising.

Our Measurements and Definitions

Baking cakes, breads, and other delectable items is a science that requires a discipline of exactness that we quite frankly do not possess. Cooking, in our opinion, should be fun and carefree. Quick and easy. And recipes should be friendly and approachable. Our recipes here are meant to offer you ideas and inspiration. If you follow them closely, you will get something delicious, but if you add to or subtract from a recipe, you will have invested in your own creativity (and that is fantastic!). As we are encouraging youth into the kitchen, we kept the recipes simple and easy. Some of our recipes do not have specific ingredients at all and are really open to your own interpretation.

Dash

"A dash" refers to one very small amount of seasoning added to food with a quick, downward stroke of the hand while holding the item's container. A dash is approximately 1/8 teaspoon and is usually a dry product. A drizzle is the same measurement for a liquid product like honey.

Splash/Drizzle

"A splash" is our term for a small amount of a liquid ingredient (such as hot sauce). It is a single but healthy squirt, or approximately 1/8 teaspoon. A "drizzle" is the term for a small amount of a thicker liquid such as maple syrup.

Pinch

"A pinch" refers to the amount of an ingredient (such as salt or pepper) that can be held between the tips of the thumb and forefinger. It too is approximately 1/8 teaspoon.

Portion Size Me-Approved Products

During our journey, we started a list of items we wanted to regularly incorporate into our household. These were store-bought items we had identified the ingredients of and basically approved of. By creating a list, we could return to these items quickly without, for example, reading all the ingredients of sandwich-bread brands every time we needed some. We considered sharing this list with you and incorporating Portion Size Me–approved products into this book, but then we realized that there are so many stores and so many brands that you may not be able to find something we are referring to. Plus, we didn't want you to spend too much time looking for products we think are good when you could be spending that time finding the brands you like in your area. That being said, we will mention a couple of items that we feel you may be able to find (or you can use our suggestions to help you look for something equivalent). We suggest that you start your own list as you begin your journey.

Our Videos

We want everyone to see Marshall's charm and inspiration during our project, so please feel free to visit our website, http://www.portionsize.me, for all the videos referenced in this book.

Please keep in mind that these videos were done with everyday technology and we have not edited them in order to keep them natural and feeling organic, the way they were created.

Our vision is not necessarily for you to follow this book from beginning to end. If you choose to, that is absolutely wonderful, but we also encourage you flip to a page or swipe to a given day and lovingly grab your child by the hand and say, "Hey, let's explore this day together." We hope that this book helps you find inspiration within yourself and your family to continue on your own healthy path.

The First Month

Bookmap

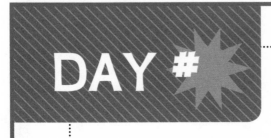

DAY #

Marshall: This is where Marshall will tell you how he is feeling each day, what he is up to, and where he wants to go on this journey.

Alex: Reflections, thoughts, and inspiration are shared here from Mom.

Recipe One

Check out these light green boxes each day for easy and healthy recipes.

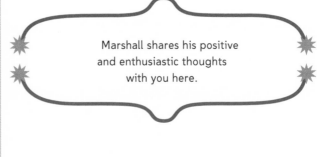

Marshall shares his positive and enthusiastic thoughts with you here.

This is where you will find quick tips and hints from Mom.

RECIPE TWO

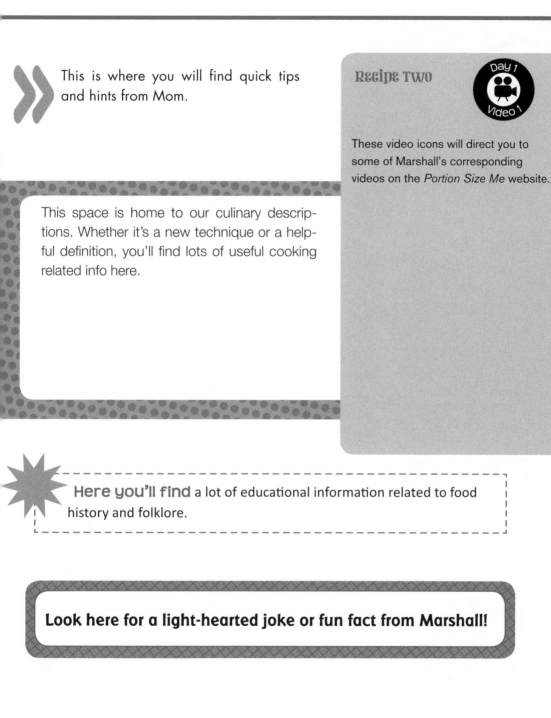

These video icons will direct you to some of Marshall's corresponding videos on the *Portion Size Me* website.

This space is home to our culinary descriptions. Whether it's a new technique or a helpful definition, you'll find lots of useful cooking related info here.

Here you'll find a lot of educational information related to food history and folklore.

Look here for a light-hearted joke or fun fact from Marshall!

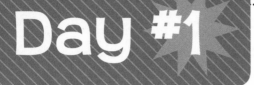

Day #1

Marshall: *I didn't start feeling different from other kids until about third grade. That's when kids started making fun of me and calling me fat. It's been constant ever since. It doesn't feel good. I want it to stop.*

Alex: I feel in many respects that I have and do set a great example for my kids in many areas, but in the consistency of dietary habits, I believe I receive a C grade. That's not a failing grade, but it certainly establishes such a wide platform for my children to base their own future eating habits on that they could easily fall for the dark side permanently. I have done well providing a wide range of variety in terms of the meals we eat, whether it's ethnic food, experimental dishes, or otherwise.

But I have shown them that in the absence of organization, planning, and time, one can still be satisfied and relatively sustained by heavily packaged and processed foods—and that is not how I want them to live.

Likewise, I have shown them that spending time in the kitchen is wonderful on special occasions, such as during the holidays, a Sunday morning brunch, or entertaining with friends. They feel good about the warmth and flavor of the kitchen, what is produced, and how it is shared. But on the flip side, I have shown them that on a daily basis, with our schedules filled with busy activities and responsibilities, the kitchen is *not* utilized as a useful tool. It is left behind in the rearview mirror as we head out to pick up a pizza.

Black and Blue Smoothie

This is where we begin to take food seriously and apply our goals. Never before has this household viewed a smoothie as anything other than a very expensive drink purchased at a restaurant and often wasted because it was overly sweetened. But now we've decided to start making our own smoothies because they are healthy, hydrating, and filling. We call this one "black and blue" because these particular berries were in season for us and we really like this combination. But feel free to use any fruit you want.

» About a cup of plain low-fat yogurt
» About a half cup of frozen blue-berries and blackberries
» A drizzle of agave nectar (this is just another natural sweetener, like honey)
» A dash of cocoa powder

Blend all ingredients in a blender.

If you want a thicker smoothie, add a couple ice cubes. If you want to go real crazy, you can add a slice of plain tofu for extra protein.

> The reason for deciding to Portion Size Me is to eat healthier and in smaller portions. First we have to start by reading labels to figure out portion sizes of things, and what's in them that is good for us and not so good for us. It is going to take a bit of time to figure all this stuff out. But we can do it!

> This is a perfect time for us to get started. It is the beginning of summer and our days are slower and longer, filled with warmth and color. We have wide windows of open time available to us instead of living in fifteen-minute increments. We need this!

Good Bugs in Your Tummy

Did you know that you have—and need—bugs in your tummy? Well, not really bugs, but rather a group of bacteria known as probiotics. They work together and create basically a chemistry lab in your digestive system, doing things such as creating hydrogen peroxide (similar to the kind you put on boo-boos), which is toxic to the bugs you don't want in your system. Eating yogurt is an easy way to replenish those good bugs that can get depleted from some medications you take or if you have been ill. It's a good idea to get your full system working in harmony again.

Diet: the collection of foods you regularly eat. Alter your collection, and you have changed your diet.

When was the last time you made a traditional BLT sandwich? Turkey bacon replaces the fattier pork variety here, and we use light mayo (or better yet, light wasabi mayo or herb mayo) on hearty Portion Size Me—approved whole-grain bread. Remember to check the ingredients of the bread you purchase. You're looking for an ingredient list that is simple and contains words you can pronounce. In our opinion, there is absolutely no reason why high-fructose corn syrup should be in your bread, as it's just an added sugar. Add thinly sliced cucumber, a few spinach leaves, lettuce, tomatoes, of course, and whatever else you have in the fridge. Thinly sliced red onion, mushrooms, parsley from the garden, and even a slice of low-fat cheese would be delicious additions. How about marinated artichoke hearts? Or our very favorite: fresh cilantro! The point here is to step away from the concept that a sandwich is boring and not satisfying. Don't make a pitiful little sandwich either. Load it up! Then give up the potato chips on the side. **Take a look at Marshall's sandwich in this video and especially pay attention to his sides!**

Marshall sat down at the kitchen table and laid it all out here on his very first video.

Day 1
Video 2

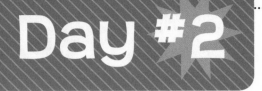
Day #2

Marshall: *I gotta tell you guys: after eating all kinds of healthy meals and foods yesterday, I feel great and I have a lot of energy. And I slept really well last night. I think it's because I put in my body more vitamins: healthier and well-balanced stuff, not just carbs but fruit and veggies. My body reacted with more energy.*

Hearty Shepherd's Pie

- » 1½ pounds lean ground beef
- » 1 onion, chopped
- » Lots of minced garlic
- » 3 large potatoes with skins on, quartered
- » Butter (just a little bit)
- » Light sour cream
- » 2 percent or skim milk
- » Salt and pepper
- » Onion powder
- » 1 package frozen sweet peas (canned sweet peas have added sugar)
- » 1 package frozen shelled edamame
- » Shredded skim Cheddar cheese

Brown beef, onion, and garlic in a skillet you can put in the oven (cast-iron cookware works great).

Boil potatoes in a pot until soft. Drain water from potatoes and mash with a tiny bit of butter, sour cream, milk, salt and pepper, and onion powder. (We paused and read the ingredients of our butter and sour cream and discovered that there was a major difference in the fat and calories between the two. So we now choose to add just a tiny bit of butter and a lot more light sour cream to our mashed potatoes. It tastes just the same to us and has the same texture as potatoes mashed with a lot more butter.)

(continued)

Alex: I feel a great sense of accomplishment when my family feels satisfied. I have spent hours in the kitchen concocting or re-creating complex recipes only to have them moan and complain. One of my early solutions to this was to inform the family that I was not altering individual plates. I was not their personal chef, and it was not my responsibility to do this for one person and that for another. I demanded that they be happy and appreciative for what they got, or they were to go hungry. How many times did I say there are starving children in other countries? But after years of trying to force them to be happy and acknowledge my efforts, I gave up. My trials to please the family in the kitchen were too great of an effort for too little of a reward. I turned to the quicker and easier meals I knew would satisfy: boxed Hamburger Helper and frozen pizzas, and as they got older, I even turned them loose in the kitchen to make their own meals of Ramen noodles and canned ravioli. Look at what I have done. How selfish of me. Marshall's summer project is a poignant reminder of where we need to get back to as a family. Let's begin!

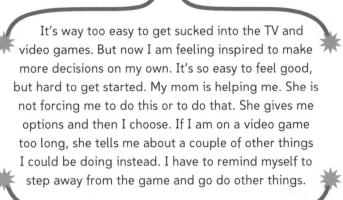

It's way too easy to get sucked into the TV and video games. But now I am feeling inspired to make more decisions on my own. It's so easy to feel good, but hard to get started. My mom is helping me. She is not forcing me to do this or to do that. She gives me options and then I choose. If I am on a video game too long, she tells me about a couple of other things I could be doing instead. I have to remind myself to step away from the game and go do other things.

Potato Myths and Truths

The potato that we take for granted has been the subject of myths, folklore, and misunderstandings. On the more fanciful side of potato mythology and folklore are several beliefs from around the world. For example, some people believe that if a pregnant woman eats potatoes, the baby will be born with a big head. In the Incan culture, the belief is that a pregnant woman who eats potatoes will have an easier childbirth. Other tales say that to cure warts, you should cut a potato in half and rub the juice on the wart. Then you can bury the potato in the ground, and as the potato rots, so will the wart.

A less extreme misunderstanding about potatoes is that they are an unhealthy diet choice. In fact, like many foods, potatoes can be very beneficial to you when they are eaten in moderation and prepared properly. Potatoes are an excellent source of vitamin C, potassium, and fiber. In fact, potatoes alone supply every vital nutrient except calcium, vitamin A, and vitamin D. The misunderstanding that potatoes are bad for you arises when salt, butter, cheese, and other things are added to potato dishes.

(continued)

Layer frozen peas and edamame on top of ground beef. Add a layer of mashed potatoes, top with a bit of Cheddar cheese, and cover.

Bake in the oven at 450°F for about 15 minutes. Then uncover and brown the cheese under the broiler.

Hearty Breakfasts Can Be Quick

A real and hearty breakfast satisfies and can be easy on busy school mornings. As quickly as you can prepare an egg, you can heat up some frozen turkey sausage, dish out a bit of fruit or yogurt, and top a slice of whole-grain bread with some marmalade. Don't be pressured to make the perfect hearty breakfast every day. Start with just twice a week. Our elementary school used to ask parents to bring in breakfast items for kids during the end-of-grade testing and ask that kids arrive early so that they could have a wonderful breakfast before they took tests. They know how important it is for kids to start their days out right. Every day is a new day! And every morning meal sets the stage for how we work and play.

Edamame is a soybean and has been eaten in Asia as a source of protein for over two thousand years. Use it shelled in lieu of corn or green beans, or eat it plain (like peanuts) after quickly boiling the beans. Edamame has a wonderful crunchy wholesomeness to it, and you can usually find the pods and beans in the grocery with other frozen vegetables.

Marshall has some great advice on making mashed potatoes for the shepherd's pie.

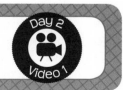

Day #3

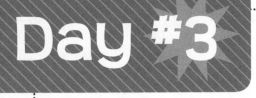

Day 3
Video 1

Chinese Crepe (Jian Bing)

» 1 cup flour (we suggest you use ½ cup white flour and ½ cup whole-wheat flour)
» 1 cup water
» 4 eggs, lightly beaten and divided (2 eggs for the batter, 2 eggs for the topping)
» Scallions, thinly sliced
» Salt
» Chili pepper sauce
» Hoisin sauce

Whisk together the flour, 2 eggs, and the water until well combined and lump free.

Spray a large skillet generously with cooking spray and heat over medium-low heat.

Pour 3 to 4 tablespoons of the batter onto the middle of the pan, and tilt the pan in a circular motion so that the batter coats the surface evenly and spreads out to make a thin crepe.

Pour the remaining 2 eggs evenly over the crepe, and then sprinkle with scallions and a pinch of salt.

Cook the pancake for about 1 to 2 minutes, until the egg is set. Flip the crepe, brush with the chili sauce and hoisin sauce, and cook for about 30 seconds. Then fold the crepe into quarters and serve. **Marshall mixes the ingredients in this video.**

Marshall: This is fun! Cooking, that is. I used to help out in the kitchen sometimes, but now I am doing a lot more. Cracking coconuts has always been my favorite kitchen activity, and for a while I thought that was all I could really do. But now I can do more, like chopping, seasoning, and even creating things. I am really enjoying it. I get to use my imagination every time I cook. We are talking a lot too about what we want to make and buy and how to be safe with food. You really have to think about everything you touch when you prepare the food. There are rules you have to follow, like washing things and using separate cutting boards for meat. It's fun spending time with my mom, and we have something to do together now because she doesn't really like to play computer games with me.

Alex: Historically, I have enjoyed the children helping in the kitchen despite the mess they make. But those occurrences have been far and few between, and it's time to start teaching the kitchen skills that will serve them throughout life. My daughter, Jordan, has created chopped concoctions for her various pet rodents and weasels and scrambled eggs for the dogs for years now. In fact, at age three or four, she would either watch Steve Irwin or the Food Network on television and nothing else. I asked her once if she wanted to be a chef when she grew up because she was watching so many cooking shows. Her response: "No, I am going to be a vet, but I have to know how to cook for my animals." Now it's time to get her thinking about fueling a human body (and learning how to clean up after herself). Marshall, being a little boy interested in all sharp, deadly objects, has confident knife skills. So it's on me to invite him into the kitchen to be the sous chef and closely monitor his progress so we don't lose any fingers in the process.

Play this game while eating a meal. You can do this by yourself or with all members of your family. Take a bite of food and try to name all the ingredients in it, including spices. To make it harder, list the ingredients from the greatest amount to the least, similar to how packaging labels are organized. This is fun, it makes you learn about different tastes, and it slows you down while eating.

Safe Food – Food Safe

The USDA recommends four basics of safe food handling: clean (hands, surfaces, food), separate (keep meats away from everything else), cook (use a thermometer to ensure you've cooked the food all the way through), and chill (don't leave things to sit out). **Watch Marshall discuss additional techniques for safely handling food.**

One province in China, Hunan, has hot, humid summers and extremely cold winters. This region is home to some of the spiciest and most flavorful dishes in the Chinese diet. It is said that the Hunan people flavor so many dishes with chilies to open the pores in their skin to keep them cool in the summer and to heat the blood in the cold winter months.

Beef Stir-Fry

Lots of fresh or frozen veggies are the winners here. Although I have had egg in fried rice at restaurants for years, I have never added it to an Asian dish made at home. Why not?

Quickly brown some lean beef chunks or strips in a large skillet with lots of garlic and a splash of sesame oil, then put aside.

Cut up lots of veggies—anything you have on hand. We used yellow squash, zucchini, mushrooms, and snow peas. You can even purchase a bag of frozen Asian vegetables. We also like to add peppers: bell peppers and a jalapeño.

Heat up your skillet with a splash of sesame oil, three splashes of soy sauce, and lots of freshly chopped garlic.

Add the veggies and cook for about 3 minutes, stirring frequently. Cook until tender but not mushy.

Add the cooked beef and three eggs, beaten with a fork.

Mix in salt and pepper, a can of water chestnuts, and another splash of soy sauce if you think you need it. You may serve this over some cooked brown rice if you wish.

Very simple, very yummy, very healthy. **Watch Marshall handle all the fresh veggies in his stir-fry.**

In *Star Trek* lingo, the second in command is called "Number One." In the military, the second in command is called the "XO." And in the kitchen, the second in command is called a sous chef. One day the parent can be the sous chef and the child can be the chef, and then you can switch the following day.

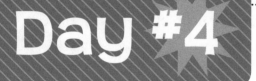

Day #4

Marshall: The point is you have to get exercise and eat healthy at the same time. You may think that exercise makes you tired, but it doesn't for some reason. Once you get more energy, you feel better and you'll eat more healthy foods. When you eat more healthy foods, you will sleep better and you'll lose weight. It's a cycle. We have been in a bad cycle, but now we are starting a good cycle.

Alex: I worry about Marshall's future. Obesity does not run on my side of the family, but it does on my husband's side. And if you are one to believe that obesity is genetic, as many scientists do, then there's at least a portion of his battle that Marshall is not responsible for. Because of my food choices I have always had an unnecessary fifteen pounds that add about one hundred pounds of insecurity. I've put up with everything from not wanting to wear bathing suits unless it's ridiculously necessary, to the careful manipulation of always being the one holding the camera to avoid someone snapping a picture of me and then being faced with viewing it. Diabetes is flirting with both sides of our family, and although I am not personally knowledgeable about how it feels to live with that disease, I do have multiple sclerosis and give myself injections several times a week. Chronic health issues are a real drag and if they can be prevented or can be lessened in their severity, I believe it is necessary to do so.

Brown Rice and Cream of Mushroom Soup

This is a recipe that Marshall created to fill himself up at lunchtime. It feels warm and satisfying, and the fiber in the brown rice makes you feel full longer. Heat a can of reduced-fat cream of mushroom soup and make as many servings of brown rice, according to the package directions, as you require. Marshall adds garlic powder and a little pepper to the soup mixture. Spoon a bit of the soup over the rice. It's quick and easy and can be made by a young one. Leftovers can easily be saved for another day—especially if you reduce your portions. Marshall has started using his fist as a visual measurement for a serving.

I get made fun of. I think it's my weight that's holding me back. I think it's my weight that's keeping me antisocial. So it's like a vicious cycle. I'm not social because I'm overweight, and I'm overweight because I'm not socially active. I just can't do the things that other kids can do. I can't go and run track. I can't play dodgeball for long periods of time, and then I am the target because I am slower. And I can't play soccer with them because I don't have the same skills. This is why I want to make changes.

Moderation is the key to many things, isn't it? How many times have we heard that or told it to others? Now I have decided to reverse that thought and think of it in this way: avoid extremes! For example, is eating this whole bag of chips extreme? Answer to yourself now, please.

Rice is a staple in the diets of over half the world's population, and it can be used in main dishes and desserts. There is fragrant rice, such as jasmine, as well as rice that is good at absorbing liquids and flavors. Actually, there are over four thousand varieties of rice, and they are all generally low in fat and a good source of vitamins and minerals. Choose a whole-grain variety and call your family to the table the way they do in Thailand by saying, "*Kin khao!*" ("Eat rice!")

chicken & whole-wheat Dumplings

I had never made this dish before now because I was always afraid that my husband would compare mine to his mothers. I know he really wouldn't, but once he was deployed, I thought it was the perfect time to give it a try and make it my own recipe.

I found some whole-wheat dumplings in the frozen pastry section of the store and thought they would be a good way to incorporate some whole grains into this rib-sticking comfort food. What I did here was incredibly easy, especially since Marshall did all the chopping.

- » Drizzle of olive oil
- » 1 serving of chicken per person
- » 1 onion, chopped
- » About 3 handfuls of celery, chopped
- » About 2 handfuls of carrots, chopped
- » Lots of fresh garlic, chopped
- » 2 cans low-fat condensed cream of chicken soup
- » 1 can condensed cream of celery soup
- » 1 package frozen whole-wheat dumplings
- » Salt & pepper

Add your olive oil to a deep skillet and begin to warm. Add chicken, onion, celery, carrots, and garlic. Cover and cook for about 10 minutes and then turn chicken and cook for another 10 minutes. Add all three cans of the soup and two cans of water. Return chicken if need be. Bring to a simmer. Now add the frozen whole-wheat dumplings. You can add them whole, but I cut mine in quarters to make them bite-sized. Salt and pepper to taste and continue to simmer for about another 10 minutes. Serve!

Rice and its by-products are used for making straw and rope, paper, wine, crackers, beer, cosmetics, packing material, and even toothpaste. It is even reported that the mortar used to hold all the huge stones together in the Great Wall of China was created from rice flour made into paste.

See Marshall talk about the importance of exercise.

Day 4
Video 1

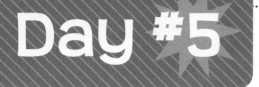

Day #5

Marshall: I've never really thought about how what goes in must go out. I mean, calories have to get burned off. If you eat too many calories, they have no place to go. If you sit there, they sit there too. Now I think of all the calories I am burning with each activity I do.

Alex: Today we went to a water park where they have wonderfully expensive hamburgers, fried chicken fingers, cotton candy, and all those exceptionally tasteful and toxic goodies. After working hard just to get the kids packed up (suits, towels, sunblock, goggles, etc.) and the car ready for the journey, it would have been very easy to just purchase the meals we needed at the water park. I reminded myself that it's on me, however, as the adult in the family, to put together a healthy picnic lunch and bypass an entire onslaught of poor eating.

Picnic Ideas

» Pre-pop some popcorn and take along individual snack-size servings. Sprinkle some lemon pepper seasoning or dried dill on the popcorn to liven it up a bit.

» Fresh whole oranges are great snacks as they are hydrating during summer heat.

» Honey sticks are super-easy travel snacks. You can find them at many farmers markets.

» Banana chips or any other dried fruits and nuts add crunch.

» Radishes are crisp and have a lot of flavor and not all of them are spicy hot. Daikon radishes are available at most grocery stores.

It's not that hard to make good food decisions when you're out and about. Like avoiding going to fast food. I mean, it can be tempting but you still have choices. Just because you're going to a fast food place doesn't mean you have to get a cheeseburger. You can get a salad. You can get apples and not eat the caramel. You can choose grilled chicken. And if you don't want to go to that kind of place, then most likely there is a grocery store close by that you can go in and buy small things like fruit, cheese, meats, and olives that you can just eat in the car. My favorite thing to do in that situation is to go into the grocery store and buy olives, sourdough bread, cheese, and olive oil. What is the American way? Stick-to-it-tiveness! That's not a real word, but you get it, don't you?

PORTION SIZE ME

One of the reasons eating out is so tasty is because restaurants load their items with tons of salt. Also, I discovered that there is a lot of sodium in sports drinks. For obvious reasons, of course, athletes have to replenish lost electrolytes. But how much salt do we wind up putting into our bodies on a daily basis? I never really thought of it.

Marshall talks about our day at the water park.
Day 5
Video 1

Watch Marshall go through snacking choices at the water park.
Day 5
Video 2

Sodium

It's elemental! The sixth most abundant element (Na) on the planet, sodium is essential for preserving foods, adding flavor, binding ingredients, and, most importantly, it is an electrolyte that every creature on the planet needs. In moderation, of course! Today there is an insurgence of gourmet salts on the market. Kosher salt, sea salt, grey salt, Hawaiian salt, and many more. Basically, these salts vary in the shape and size of the granule. Some grains are large, and others are tiny, round, and smooth. One might also choose a salt based on its origin, lending to a subtle flavor experience.

The Food and Nutrition Board of the National Academy of Sciences estimates that an "adequate and safe" intake of sodium for healthy adults is 1,100 to 3,300 milligrams a day, the equivalent of approximately ½ to 1½ teaspoons of salt. That is a fairly wide range. But keep in mind that a few slices of pizza can scale 2,300 milligrams in sodium—and that is just one meal.

Day #6

Day 6
Video 2

Grilled Turkey Breasts with Sweet Potatoes and Pineapple

» ½ sweet potato per serving
» 1 boneless, skinless turkey breast per serving (or you can use chicken, if you prefer)
» 1 whole fresh pineapple for many servings
» Salt and pepper

Light your grill or coals.

Rinse the sweet potato and slice it into ½-inch thick slices, leaving the skin on. Place the potato slices on the grill while you prepare the turkey breast and season it with salt and pepper.

To prepare the pineapple, cut either end off. Then stand it on one end and slice the outer skin off all the way around. If the pineapple is nice and ripe, you can leave the core in. Otherwise, cut it into quarters and then slice the end with the core off.

Put the turkey breasts on the grill, and place a slice of pineapple on top of each piece of turkey. Turn the turkey and sweet potato in about 5 minutes, and place the pineapple back on top of the turkey. When the potatoes are soft and the turkey is cooked through, place the pineapple slices on the hottest part of the grill and brown them.

The cool thing about this dish is that everything gets put on the grill, so there are no pots and pans to clean up.

Watch Marshall prep a pineapple for this recipe.

Marshall: I am just tired of sitting around and doing the same old thing. What I have been doing has not been working for me, so I wanna change it. I want to go everywhere and do everything. Now I am going to focus on developing three areas: my strength, agility, and speed. At sixteen, I want to feel good and look slim, not as bulky. I think I may want to run a marathon when I am eighteen. I want to feel strong and be able to run with my friends and have fun with them and not have to check my blood sugar every ten minutes. At age forty, I want to be able to keep up on the house and fix the car. I don't want to be weighed down by hurting limbs because I'm too large for them to hold me.

Alex: Most of us do not have an intimate knowledge of and relationship with food the way previous generations had. No more do we plan our days around sustaining our food sources and fueling our families, building relationships with neighbors over hunted meats, harvesting our crops, and preserving foods for the winter season.

Today, our attention is turned to clocks and schedules: work, traffic, banking, school, soccer, T-ball. It seems as if food and nutrition have been reduced to a level of importance even lower than deciding upon the clothes we wear to accomplish our daily tasks. For some, food has become the comfort needed to face those scheduled lifestyles instead of the nourishing fuel to power the human body. Now, food not only has to provide nutrients, but it is also given the job of helping us cope and emotionally get through the day. That's a big responsibility to place on proteins, grains, vegetables, and such.

I have noticed that Marshall has begun eating out of boredom, and that will only continue into adulthood if we allow food to be solely comfort food. I must preserve the wholesome bond that sitting around the dinner table creates and reintroduce my family members to traditions we once shared that lead to healthy behaviors despite the tick-tock nature of our lives.

> You really need to keep on your parents to get out and play with you. It's easy for them to tell you to go play, but they can play with you too some of the time. So ask them to join you!

»» For children who have never been around a grill, or younger children you are just introducing to grilling, you may consider picking up a mini-grill or using a Sterno like we did with these meatballs. It's less daunting, and children can move around it more safely.

Frying versus Grilling

There is pan-frying, shallow-frying, and deep-fat frying. In order, these involve a little bit of oil, a medium amount of oil, and a whole heck of a lot of oil. Some suggest that frying a product that does not absorb the oil, such a skinless chicken, is not too bad for you. But cooking something that can absorb the oil, such as the skin on chicken or breading, significantly increases the oil content you eat. Grilling is a dry-heat cooking method, but that doesn't mean the item has to be dry. Add a sauce and it could be called a barbeque. Grilling is generally considered healthier than frying because there is not as much oil absorbed into the food. However, you can still do some damage to calorie and fat content when grilling something such as chicken with its skin coated in a buttery, sugary sauce.

Charcoal absorbs and holds moisture, so make sure you store it in a dry place.

Astronaut cabbage

Cut the base of a whole cabbage so it sits upright without rolling over. Remove any loose or discolored outer leaves. Place a Sterno can on the top and use a knife to trace around the Sterno, scoring a mark in the cabbage. Now, using a paring knife, cut lines within the circle you have just created and gently remove the cabbage in that circle. Work your way deeper and deeper until enough cabbage is removed that you can insert the Sterno can flush with the top of the cabbage. (These portable cooking-fuel containers can be found in the camping section or cooking section of many retailers. As an aside, these handy Sternos are great to keep in your home emergency kit.)

Cut bamboo skewers to varying sizes.

Either prepare lean meatballs and fully cook them or purchase and heat frozen cooked turkey meatballs. Stick a meatball on one end of a skewer, and place the other end of the skewer into the cabbage. Fill up the whole cabbage with skewers so it looks fun and crazy—like something from outer space.

Provide dipping sauces for the meatballs, such as wasabi, mustards, or sweet and sour sauce.

To eat, pull a skewer with a meatball from the cabbage, warm it over the Sterno, and dip it in the sauce. This is fun anytime, and don't worry, Sternos are used by professional cooks all the time and are quite safe. **See what it looks like in this video.**

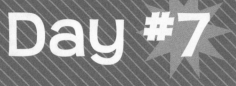

Day #7

Small Steps Quiche

This recipe makes two quiche pies: one for dinner and one for breakfast. This is a great recipe to get kids involved with, or for a child to make on Mother's Day!

- » ½ chopped onion
- » Lots of minced garlic
- » 1 pound cubed ham, turkey, or chicken
- » 1 package fresh mushrooms
- » 1 pound fresh asparagus
- » 2 frozen deep-dish pie crusts
- » 1 cup light Monterey Jack cheese, divided
- » 8 eggs
- » 1½ cups milk
- » 1 tablespoon whole-wheat flour

Add onion, garlic, ham, mushrooms, and asparagus to a pan and cook over high heat for about 10 minutes, stirring frequently.

Follow the directions for the frozen pie crusts, and add ½ cup of cheese to the bottom of each crust.

Whisk the eggs, milk, and flour in medium bowl. Add half of the ham mixture to each pie. It should fill about three-quarters of the pie shell. Pour half of the egg mixture over the ham mixture in each pie. Bake at 350°F for about 35 minutes.

You can of course add salt and pepper to the egg mixture if you wish, and you can garnish the quiches with sliced fresh tomatoes and cilantro if you want.

Marshall: Try to make your lifestyle changes in small little steps. If you're making a hamburger, don't completely cut out the beef and replace it with other leaner meats all at once. Just add a little leaner meat each time you make it. Try not to do everything at once. Do it in small steps. A good example of leaner meat is turkey. Most of the time it is leaner than beef and it can make it taste even better. My friend Teddy Herra rode his bicycle around the country, and I asked him how he was doing it. He said, "One pedal at a time." That's what we're saying here. If you leap and don't take small steps, you are sure to fall.

Meet Teddy and watch him talk about his journey.

Day 7 Video 1

Alex: It's not easy making changes, and getting the family on board with the Portion Size Me routine isn't any easier. First, we are learning, and that takes energy. And we all know that when our energy levels feel strained, we really don't want to put out any more effort—we want to slip back into comfortable patterns. With three of us here (my husband is deployed overseas), we don't have taxed energy levels at the same time. Sometimes when Jordan is feeling positive and cooperative, Marshall is down, mumbling and stomping his feet. Once we get the hang of this, it will be time for my husband to get home, and then we will have to help him make small changes.

If someone gives you food and you don't know what the ingredients are, just take a small serving and add something healthy on the side to balance it out. My Aunt Pepper (that's her nickname) brought over some quiche one day. We were pretty sure she added a lot of butter and cream to it too, because she likes to go all out on things like that.

Watch Marshall and Jordan balance out Aunt Pepper's quiche with a healthy option.

Day 7 Video 2

PORTION SIZE ME

Our Simple Kitchen Lingo

Beat: to stir rapidly in a circular motion by hand, about one hundred strokes per minute

Mix: to combine things together, usually with an electric beater

Stir/Blend: to combine things with a spoon

Fold: a way to combine things very gently, usually using a flat spatula or rubber spatula, scooping from the bottom and folding the mixture over the top

Whip: to mix at high speed, usually with an electric beater

Pancakes with Blueberries and Dark Chocolate Chips

Studies come and go as quickly as the sun rises and falls. Currently, dark-chocolate is considered good for you. But that doesn't mean that it's OK to eat six dark chocolate candy bars a day. These pancakes have moderation written all over them. Add just a few dark chocolate chips and a few healthy frozen blueberries to your preferred pancake recipe. Also, many pancake recipes call for white flour so you may consider mixing it half white flour and half wheat or buckwheat flour. We also choose to use real maple syrup instead of the heavily processed kind. It is more expensive, but a little goes a long way. Honestly, I don't even use any syrup on these pancakes—they're delicious on their own. The melted chocolate and warm blueberries are rich and wonderful. These small choices really add up over time!

The Native Americans taught the colonists how to tap the maple tree for its sap and boil it down to what the Native Americans called "sweetwater." The "sugar makers" insert spouts into the maple trees and hang buckets from them to catch the sap. Sometimes plastic tubing is connected to the spout, running from tree to tree and eventually directly to a large holding tank where it's stored until it's ready to be processed. The sap is then taken to the "sugarhouse," where it's boiled until thickened to the desired degree. Quite simply, maple syrup is sap that has been boiled until much of the water has evaporated and the sap is thick and syrupy. At the beginning of the syrup season, when the sap is concentrated, it only takes about twenty gallons of it to make one gallon of syrup, but at the end of the season, it may take up to fifty gallons.

Small choices: if your body is well-balanced between food and exercise, and you add just one soda a day for a year while continuing your healthy regime, you will gain fourteen pounds. Conversely, what changes will happen to you if you cut out your soda?

Track

Mom's Quick Tip!
What are some of the healthy things you already enjoy? List them here to make sure that you remember them and keep them in your diet collection.

Your Journey!

Helpful Hint:

Um, you might be surprised by this, but one of my new favorite snacks is a bell pepper. The green ones are OK, but the yellow and the red ones are sweeter. I eat them just like you eat an apple. And my mom buys those mini peppers and they are really, really good. Try some...and make sure you wash them first!

Track

Mom's Quick Tip!

One example of small choices that can add up and make an impact over time is the house rule we created to stand up while playing the Wii. I think it also reminds you how long you are actually playing when your legs and back get tired.

Your Journey!

Helpful Hint:

Always remember to check your ingredients! It's OK to use premade items if you check the label and understand what's in it. It can help you make meals more quickly and simply and explore new flavors. For example, we really like Thai Kitchen Green Curry Paste, and it is *Portion Size Me*–approved!

Day #8

Hummus

Fresh hummus is a good source of iron, folate, and the vitamins C and B6. In addition, the chickpeas provide protein and fiber. When you add the tahini, you add methionine, a necessary amino acid.

This is Jordan's recipe and about her favorite thing to make. Taste your way through preparing this dish, adding more or less of the ingredients to make it the way you like it. You can also add ingredients such as roasted red peppers or capers, Jordan's favorite.

By the way, you can usually find tahini in the peanut butter section or ethnic food aisle of the grocery store. After eating this hummus as a dip, the next day you can make a Mediterranean wrap using the hummus in lieu of mayo. Just add some feta cheese, salad greens, and olives in a wrap. Mmmm!

- » 4 cans garbanzo beans (chickpeas), drained
- » 3 tablespoons tahini
- » Lots and lots of fresh garlic
- » 2 tablespoons lemon juice
- » Splash of olive oil
- » Salt and pepper
- » Assorted veggies, wheat crackers, or slices of wheat pita

Place all the ingredients in a food processor or blender. Blend until the ingredients are a smooth consistency. Serve with the veggies, wheat crackers, or pita.

Marshall: To me, "healthy" means eating real foods, having the right amount of exercise, and not being so overweight that you cannot run. I am on the edge of being like that. Healthy means that you need to not be overweight. That's really my main goal, to get out of the overweight category and eat more real foods, instead of all the easy junk you can buy at the store just because it's cheap. Eating healthy might be a little bit expensive, but it will really help you in the long run.

Alex: It is so easy to fall into the trap of ending the argument as quickly as possible. For me, that often means not getting what I want or need done from Marshall. It is so easy to get sucked into arguing rather than establishing limits or consequences. Marshall is so intelligent and such a good communicator (read: "argues quite well") that I get baited. I forget that he is so young, that he lacks complex maturity, and that he *does* require boundaries and limits. I set restrictions and boundaries in other areas, including bedtime, homework, chores, and general manners and behaviors, but eating properly and respecting food has escaped me. For example, snacking. My kids have been allowed to grab a juice box and a snack anytime they want. The result of not having boundaries about only snacking at a certain time has been too many calories being taken in and not getting burned off.

> You have got to establish good habits for eating, just like you do for sleeping and brushing your teeth.

How do you define "healthy"? Is it a picture in a magazine? Something you want to be able to do, such as join a recreational team? Avoiding high blood sugar or type 2 diabetes? Anyway you define it, don't try to get there all at once. Healthy doesn't happen overnight. But it can start right now and be a part of every decision you make.

Good Acids For You!

Of the twenty-two different amino acids, there are eight essential amino acids that your body can only get from the food that you eat. Some foods, such as animal products, have all eight amino acids to make the protein you receive complete. Many plant foods, such as beans, have only some of the amino acids. By eating more than one incomplete amino acid plant-based meal, you can gain all eight that you need. Protein is vital to every aspect of your body, from muscle development to digestion and metabolism. And it is not affected by lower calorie choices, such as reduced-fat milk or cheese, because the protein is still there in the food even if the calories are not.

Cuban Black Beans

- » 1 package dry black beans
- » 4 servings ham (you can use leftovers from a whole cooked ham, ham steaks, or cubed ham)
- » 1 onion, chopped
- » 1 green bell pepper, chopped
- » Lots of whole garlic cloves, sliced or chopped
- » Dash of cumin
- » Salt and pepper
- » Fresh cilantro, chopped
- » Hot sauce, such as Tabasco
- » Cooked brown rice

Follow the directions on the package to cook the beans. If you can throw a ham bone into the water with the beans, that will make them extra flavorful.

Brown the ham with the onion, bell pepper, and garlic in a pan on the stove. Add to the cooked beans, and then add the cumin, salt, and pepper to taste.

Serve with cilantro and hot sauce over brown rice. Yum!

Peanuts, soybeans, and beans are in the same family as thousands of other plants that have seed pods that split along both sides when ripe. These are called legumes. Legumes are high in fiber and B vitamins.

You get exercise from a wide variety of fun activities. Watch Marshall exercise while at the driving range.

Day 8
Video 1

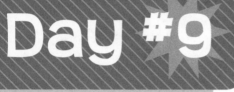

Day #9

Green Curry with Snow Peas and Artichokes

This is super quick and easy, thanks to the wonderful flavors of Thai Kitchen Green Curry Paste and the delightful tang of artichoke hearts. If you want to get your kids in the kitchen but they don't yet have knife skills, try having them perform other kitchen tasks, such as tenderizing the meat.

» Jasmine rice
» Lean beef or chicken cut into bite-size pieces
» Chopped onion
» Lots of garlic
» 1 can light coconut milk
» 1 package frozen snow peas
» 1 can artichoke hearts, chopped
» Fresh or canned pineapple chunks
» 1 tablespoon, or more, Thai Kitchen Green Curry Paste
» Fresh cilantro

Cook the jasmine rice according to the directions on the package.

Brown the meat in a deep skillet with the onion and garlic.

Add the remaining ingredients and simmer, covered, for about 10 to 12 minutes. (You don't want to overcook the snow peas.) Add more green curry paste if you like, but a little goes a long way.

Spoon the meat and vegetable mixture over the rice. (Or, if your kids don't like their food to touch, like one of my munchkins, serve the rice on the side.) Add a touch of water if you want more sauce, and garnish with fresh cilantro.

Marshall: I am enjoying cooking. My favorite part is tasting the dishes when they are done! I like cooking with my mom because I don't have to do everything by myself; you know there is somebody with you. I like cutting up all the ingredients we use. It takes skill, but it's fun too. You have to know where to cut it and how to cut it, what angle to cut it and how much to cut off. You don't just randomly chop around.

Alex: I am really quite surprised and happy that Marshall has continued with Portion Size Me (PSM). He really seems to enjoy being in front of the camera. I think one of the best things about this is that Marshall is learning from teaching. I know I make better choices when I am in a role model position, and I actually learn more from teaching than being taught. I think this is the same for Marshall.

What can you do in your family to put your children in teaching situations so that they can learn from the teaching experience? Since we are talking about getting back into the kitchen and eating real foods, can you have your older child teach a younger sibling how to make a healthy meal? Or can you have your children go through the pantry cabinet, reading the labels of canned food? Or ask them to find all the hidden sugars on your canned products in your kitchen. Ask them to do a demonstration for you, like Marshall's videos, of what they found. Put the camera on them and see what they come up with!

>> Our family likes to host themed dinner parties, and guests are required to bring dishes in line with the theme. We've covered the basics, with Mexican night and Chinese night, and then we've delved even deeper. We hosted a Kenyan night and a Saudi Arabian night, where we even dressed up and sat on pillows in the living room. This was great fun, with

many hours of entertainment, and most importantly, it introduced new foods to the kids. Today, they have a wide-ranging palate, I think in part to our wonderful dinner parties.

What theme-based dinner parties can you come up with? Or even better, task your children to come up with a plan. You don't have to do this every week or even every month. Trying it just once can open up new horizons for those little taste buds.

Sometimes I get a little bit mad at myself when I do something wrong. But you're always going to do something a little wrong. It's impossible not to. Like my mom really didn't like it that I was using expensive paintballs to shoot from my slingshot. But hey, I was outside trying to keep my body moving. Even when you're cooking in the kitchen, you may do something wrong. But does it really matter that you chopped something instead of diced it? Will the world end? Unless you burn it or over-salt it, what's the harm? I'm trying to say not to be too hard on yourself when you make a mistake. All things seem harder when you stress over it.

Marshall gets clever with his activities.

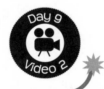

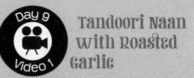

Tandoori Naan with Roasted Garlic

Many stores now carry a large variety of ethnic foods. We found another PSM–approved product from Trader Joe's: tandoori naan. I have also seen naan at other stores. Naan is an Indian flatbread baked on the walls of a tandoori oven. You can find it in the frozen section and sometimes in the bakery section, and it only takes minutes to prepare with the directions on the package. If you can't find naan, you can substitute whole-wheat pita bread.

We like to spread roasted garlic on top of our naan. Take an elephant garlic clove and cut the top off of it, just exposing the little tips of each clove; wrap it in foil; and drizzle a little bit of olive oil on it. Bake it in the oven for about 20 minutes at 400°F, and then spread the warm, soft garlic over your naan like butter.

Check out Marshall as he prepares naan with garlic.

The process of preserving foods, like the coconut milk and artichoke hearts in our green curry recipe, was invented in 1809. The tin can was born to do so. But there was one problem! The cans had to be broken into, because the can opener was not invented until almost fifty years later.

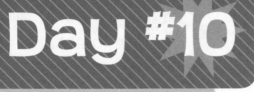

Day #10

Angel Hair & Yogurt

I made this by accident once when I was poor and in school in NYC. All I had was pasta and plain yogurt. I thought perhaps the yogurt would make a type of alfredo sauce. And although that idea didn't quite work out, as alfredo sauce has a lot of cheese in it, I enjoyed this so much that I actually played around with ways to keep the yogurt cool against the hot noodles. That was very appealing to me, having two different temperatures in one bite. This recipe is SO simple you won't have to spend too much time reading labels and checking the quality of ingredients. You only need two things: whole-wheat angel hair pasta and low-fat plain yogurt (even Greek yogurt will do). Follow the directions of the package to cook the noodles, being extra careful not to overcook them. Then, with tongs, remove the amount you want from the hot water and quickly put into a bowl. Add a couple of spoonfuls of yogurt and maybe a pinch of salt. Now don't mix the yogurt completely through the noodles. Leave it as spoonfuls on top of your hot noodles and just pass your noodles on your fork through the yogurt before you take a bite. This allows the yogurt to not get overheated from the noodles. The nuttiness from the noodles and tanginess from the yogurt, combined with the temperature differences, really is unique.

Marshall: Nobody ever cares to look at the label. Companies seem to hide things in their products, things like high-fructose corn syrup (HFCS), sugars, extra fats. But not always are the things hiding in the food bad for you—you could get vitamins, minerals, and other things that could end up helping you. But most of the time you get those things that are just to make the food easier to mass produce cheaply. Before I started this I never looked at labels, but now I do and I think the reason that I didn't read labels before was because I just didn't care and didn't think it mattered. I thought everything was just like it seemed. And a lot of the time the fine print is extremely fine and I think that's cheap; they don't want people to see what they are saying.

Alex: High-fructose corn syrup and monosodium glutamate (MSG) are examples of products with scientific research on either side of the fence, meaning you can find scientists that say that these products are harmful and scientists that say they are not harmful. You can find groups and organizations' marketing communications saying they are fine, and other groups and organizations spending marketing money to say they are harmful. What are you to possibly believe? Well, here are my honest thoughts on flavor enhancers added to your packaged foods. Why are they even needed? Those items themselves are heavily processed or genetically modified, and I don't care to have them in my body. See, now I don't even have to watch the commercials anymore about one side or the other. I've just decided for myself.

We left some space in these pages for you to start a list of healthy items you like and recipes you like. It's easy to forget stuff. But if you get hungry and need an idea, you can go to the list you made in this book and remind yourself of what you liked.

PORTION SIZE ME

Are Calories Our Enemies?

"Calorie" has become a household word, although exactly what a calorie does is a mystery to many. Calories have gotten a bad reputation and are considered by many to be the enemy. Few people truly understand what a calorie is and why it is so important to their bodies. Calories are the energy that fuels our bodies, much like gasoline fuels our cars. Without sufficient calories, our hearts would not beat, our lungs would not function, and our brains would not work. If you exceed the number of calories your body requires each day, you will eventually gain weight.

It's important to remember that although drastically reducing your calories in a short period of time may initially result in dramatic weight loss, the body can rarely continue along this restrictive path.

Monosodium Glutamate (MSG), a flavor enhancer, is added to a wide variety of foods, from Chinese food, fried chicken, and luncheon meats to sauces and spices. It can also be labeled as hydrolyzed protein yeast extract, sodium caseinate, textured protein, or glutamic acid. MSG was discovered by a chemist in 1908, and it was so popular that the Japanese coined it *umami*, translating in English to "savory." Some people claim to feel overly fatigued and to suffer from headaches after eating food products with MSG, while an entire country has used it harmlessly for decades.

See how Marshall feels after eating Chinese food with MSG in it.

Day 10
Video 1

Homemade Ketchup

From a dipping sauce to hot-wing sauce to cocktail sauce, ketchup is a common household staple that wears many hats. Let's make our own today! If it's summertime, you'll probably find that tomatoes are plentiful.

» 7 cups tomatoes, chopped
» 1 yellow onion, chopped
» 2 cloves garlic, chopped
» 1 celery stalk, chopped
» 1 red bell pepper, seeds removed and chopped
» 2 tbsp. dark brown sugar
» ½ cup cider vinegar
» 1 cup water
» Pinch cayenne
» Pinch celery salt
» Pinch dry mustard
» Pinch ground allspice
» Pinch ground cloves
» Pinch ground ginger
» Pinch ground paprika
» Pinch ground cinnamon
» Salt and pepper to taste
» Cornstarch on the side if you need to thicken the ketchup after cooking

Add all the ingredients to a heavy-duty stock pot. Stir well and bring to a boil.

Simmer, stirring regularly, for about an hour and a half. The reason for cooking so long is to break down the contents and reduce it (meaning to evaporate the water).

Blend the contents of the stock pot in a blender really well. Season to taste.

Depending on the types of tomatoes you used, you may have to add a pinch or two of cornstarch to thicken it to your liking.

Day #11
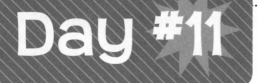

Marshall: The colors at the farmers' market are extremely beautiful. It's nice to see all of the colors next to each other all at once. Just piles and piles of fruits and vegetables and homemade treats like bread and cheese. Looking at all the different foods is guaranteed to make your mouth water. So good! They sell little straws filled with honey at the market, and they are so sweet they make your eyes fill with joy. We buy a few of them and add them to my lunch box. They are OK to eat because the honey is natural and from local bees. Try your best to support local farmers because most likely, they won't try to hide stuff in complicated ingredients. If it's not good, they won't sell it to you.

Alex: I encourage you to go out and spend time at local farmers' markets. The easiest way to find them is to simply do a Google search for markets in your area. There is a fabulous site called LocalHarvest.org where you enter your ZIP code to locate farmers' markets close to you. Another option is to call your local agricultural extension office. We have a little local farmers' market, and then we have the big state-fair farmers' market about forty-five minutes away. The kids really enjoy going.

Watch Jordan at our local market.

Marshall's Barley Stew (otherwise known as Mulligan Stew)

Boil enough water for your serving size. Add lean stewing beef. Add beef bouillon according to the amount of water you used. Boil for 5 minutes. Add diced celery, diced carrots, chopped onion, lots of whole garlic cloves, and a little barley. Boil 10 minutes more, or for as long as the package directions specify to cook the barley. Remove from heat and let cool for 5 minutes. Then eat up!

Marshall makes barley stew.

I used to snack on potato chips a lot, but to tell you the truth, right now I prefer peaches. Peaches are 100 percent real, as long as you don't buy a canned version that has high-fructose corn syrup.

I didn't grow up in a household that bought food in bulk and saved every bit of it. We purchased only what was needed and used it. I also didn't have grandparents who showed me how they grew up during the Depression or with wartime rationing. Now I am married to a farm boy from Iowa, and I see how his family has multiple freezers and nothing is wasted. One family member still has that "waste nothing" mentality in regards to items on sale at the grocery store. His huge freezers—yes, plural on "freezers"—are filled to capacity at all times. It's occurring to me now to find the balance between freezing some of these glorious items found at the farmers' market and stuffing my freezer to an unusable capacity. Frozen bananas are a fun item to keep for later. Use them to make banana bread.

Why So Cold?

Freezing preserves food quality, but it does not improve it, so freeze foods at the peak of their ripeness. If the item or dish you are freezing contains an acidic ingredient, like tomatoes, cover it first with plastic wrap and then heavy aluminum foil. There can be a reaction between the food and the foil that's distasteful. Keep in mind too that some items, like green beans, corn, and zucchini, require blanching (boiling very quickly in water and then placing into an ice bath) prior to freezing. This is an important step because it destroys enzymes that would reduce the quality of the food and could make it taste poorly after freezing. My new go-to produce to freeze is bananas. I then use them later to make banana bread.

Fruity Grilled Chicken Wings

These super easy wings can be cooked on a grill or under the broiler. And here is an opportunity to use some fresh preserves you may have found at a local farmers' market. I call them "fruity" wings because most preserves or jams are made from fruit, but you can also use local hot-pepper jellies or chow chows (the sweet or sour pickled vegetables you find in the pickle section of the grocery store). Generously coat the chicken wings (and drumsticks too, if you'd like) with your local preserved product, then place them on the grill or under the broiler. Keep in mind that many jams and preserves are full of sugar, so you can cut fat by taking the skin off the wings and using the preserves to make a crispy, candied coating. It's a give and take: since there is a little extra sugar in this meal, we will try to have a little less fat by removing the skin.

Believe it or not, frozen food has a long history. It has been popular since 3,000 BCE, when the ancient Chinese used ice cellars to preserve food through cold winter months. The Romans also used to store food in compressed snow in insulated cellars. The Food and Drug Administration has confirmed that frozen fruits and vegetables provide the same essential nutrients and health benefits as fresh. That makes sense. Frozen fruits and vegetables are nothing more than fresh fruits and vegetables that have been picked at their ripest, cooked for a short time in boiling water or by being steamed, and then frozen.

Marshall enjoys riding his bike – a great way to get exercise!

Day 11
Video 3

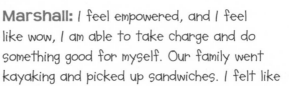

Day #12

Marshall: I feel empowered, and I feel like wow, I am able to take charge and do something good for myself. Our family went kayaking and picked up sandwiches. I felt like I was the leader of the pack because I had the responsibility to make sure we got the right chips with the sandwiches and that they were good for us. I feel like I am my own person and not a robot. I feel like I can make my own decisions and not have everyone tell me you can only eat this or you can only eat that. It's a great feeling when you do something good.

Watch my family as we kayak and see the food decisions we made.

Grilled Cherries

Simple, yummy, and fun, grilling fruits is wonderful in the summertime, or during the spring or fall. Throw some fresh fruit on the grill whenever you are finished with making a meal, and use the leftover heat to make a wonderful dessert. Something about the heat brings out more flavors in the fruit. We have done this with whole cherries and sliced, fresh pineapple, and we have even tried orange slices on the grill. Go ahead and experiment. Just wash and dry your fruit first. If you eat a fruit whole with the skin on, then leave it that way. If you generally remove the skin or slice a piece of fruit, go ahead and do that. Make sure your grill is cleaned with a wire brush first. And don't bother the fruit too much by constantly turning it. It may begin to fall apart. Use a spatula instead of tongs. Lastly, if your fruit gets too soft or if it is so small it falls through the grill, try putting it on top of a piece of aluminum foil.

Marshall makes grilled cherries.

Alex: The other day, we ate out and I was happy to note some of the choices the kids made on their own. Marshall did not go straight for the mac and cheese: he had various salads first, and then hit the mac and cheese. The piece of that example that stands out to me the most is that he is beginning to consciously think about food, building a healthy relationship with it and beginning to make decisions on his own. I am very proud of him and Jordan for being open to these new ideas. This can only end up positively.

You want to sort of push away the bad stuff and bring in the new stuff! Take the time to investigate what you are eating. Try trading out potato chips for fresh fruit, or a Twinkie for a handful of nuts. It's the snacking that really works against me, but a piece of fruit, like an apple, takes time to eat and doesn't go down as quick as a piece of string cheese. That choice makes me more satisfied.

Have a young tadpole wanting to grill with you but perhaps you're concerned they will get hurt around a large, hot grill? Start out by putting the beautiful food in or on a piece of aluminum foil. It is really hard to burn something in aluminum, and it keeps the flames from reaching up and licking at any juices coming from the food. Also, it's a larger surface that foods can be moved around on, which does not require fully developed fine-motor skills, and the little ones will have success, which is the point after all. Another option is to purchase a mini-grill; ours is a little terra-cotta pig. You can find them in all shapes and configurations these days at local hardware stores and local greenhouses or garden centers. It's hard to knock over, and kids can reach all the way around it instead of accidentally leaning on a hot grill. Consider even having the bulk of your grilling foods on the main grill while supervising the little one with their own mini-grill.

Traditional Latkes

Latkes are delightful potato pancakes. Crispy on the outside and soft and warm in the middle, these traditional Jewish celebratory pancakes can now be readily found boxed in many grocery stores. I have read the packaging of a lot of different brands, and the ingredients look wholesome despite the food being packaged. These little gems are supposed to be deep fried, but I have discovered that a light drizzle of olive oil in a nonstick skillet works fabulously, and they can be make quickly for busy school mornings. Give it a try! You can also try using leftover mashed potatoes and make your own latkes, although I find I have to use a lot of oil in the pan and sear them really quickly to hold them together.

Currently, the USDA does not have specific guidelines on how many antioxidants one should consume. But cherries are always a good choice if you're trying to get more anti-oxidants, which are nutrients in our food that strengthen our immune systems. Scientists believe eating a diet rich in antioxidants is a proactive antidote to fighting off some serious diseases, like cancer, in the future.

Did you know that avocados and olives are fruits? Technically, if something contains seeds, then it is a fruit. It is the fruit of a flowering plant from which it grows.

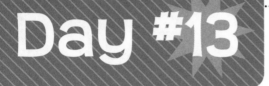

Day #13

Marshall: Let's talk cravings. I think I have been able to deal with some of them. I say, "Hold on, Marshall; do you really need this, or is it another stupid craving?" The only reason I say "stupid" is because they are annoying. They will not leave me alone. I like to say, "Step aside, craving. I don't like you." Sometimes if I am craving a vanilla milkshake, I will just go and have a cup of milk. That's it.

Alex: I was sitting talking to my friend, Terri, one day about this project, and she blurted out, "I'm guilty of it!" "Guilty of what?" I asked. She described the issue of rewarding her son by feeding into and satisfying his sugar cravings. Now, Terri is a very healthy and fit person and works hard to make sure her son eats well too. She continued and asked me, "Why can't I reward him with healthy treats? Why are the fresh, good things not the reward?" Then she said, "Unless it's strawberries from Gross Farms." "What?" I asked. "Because Adam remembers going to the farm and picking strawberries, so if I just swing by and pick some up without making it a strawberry-picking event, he still loves them like they are a special treat." My take on that conversation was that an experience, an event, a tradition can change one's viewpoint. That's what we are trying to learn here and make happen more consistently in our lives. We can change the way we view our "treats" by incorporating more "real food" experiences.

Make Your Own Burrito

To me, a burrito is just a vessel. You can put anything you want in it. I like to bite into something like this and experience a warm temperature followed by the crisp, cool freshness of lettuce or cilantro and a tang of lime. It tells my mind that there is a lot going on.

- » 1 can fat-free refried beans or whole black beans, drained
- » Brown rice (You can find brown rice in individual servings that you can microwave. It's a waste from a packaging perspective, but quite handy for something like this.)
- » Whole-wheat tortilla
- » Salsa
- » Low-fat shredded cheese
- » Low-fat sour cream
- » Fresh cilantro, minced
- » Dash of cumin
- » Lots of garlic, minced
- » Squeeze of lime juice

Heat the beans and rice in the microwave, and then spread them onto the tortillas.

Top with the remaining ingredients. Be careful not to overload the burritos, because they will be too hard to fold. Feel free to add more items from your fridge, including sliced cabbage, chopped peppers, diced onion, and maybe even some leftover green curry from Day 9. Fold and heat in microwave again.

You can also make several burritos at once, and once they are completely cooled, wrap them in plastic wrap, then aluminum foil, and freeze them for individual meals. To reheat from frozen, just unwrap the burritos and let them sit out at room temperature until defrosted. Then wrap them in paper towel and microwave on high for about 3 minutes.

stuffed cabbage

Like the tortilla of the burrito, the cabbage here is just a vessel to hold the yummy ingredients.

- » 1 head green cabbage
- » 1 pound or more of lean ground beef (or half beef and half lean ground turkey)
- » 1 onion, diced
- » Lots of fresh chopped garlic
- » Salt and pepper
- » Dash of oregano
- » Cooked brown rice for 6 servings (we are making a pan for leftovers)
- » 2 cans diced or stewed tomatoes with juice
- » ½ cup to ¾ cup grated Asiago cheese (or any cheese you'd like; Parmesan is my next favorite)

Throw the whole head of cabbage in the microwave and cook for about 5 minutes at a time. Let it cool for 1 or 2 minutes, and then gently peel off the outer leaves as gently as you possibly can. Try to peel them so that the leaves remain whole. Repeat until you have as many whole leaves as you need. Do not discard the remaining cabbage head; I have a suggestion below for it.

Brown the meat with the onion, garlic, salt, pepper, and oregano in a large skillet, breaking the meat into small pieces with a fork.

Add the rice and tomatoes; stir and simmer for about 10 minutes. Taste your mixture and make sure you're happy with it.

Add a spoonful of the mixture to the base of each leaf, and carefully roll the leaf. Place in a baking dish.

After you have filled one baking dish, you'll notice you have a lot more mixture. You can make another pan of rolls or do it the lazy way I do. I just take the remaining cabbage head and shred it. Then I layer the shredded cabbage and filling in another baking dish.

Sprinkle the grated Asiago cheese lightly over the top of your pans, and bake at 400°F, covered, for about 20 minutes.

Mise en place simply means to have everything out and in place before you start cooking. It's practical and safe to spend a moment to ensure you are prepared. It's not entirely necessary to go as far as to premeasure everything and put the ingredients in little bowls, like you see on the TV cooking shows, but it is *fun*!

Also referred to as roughage, dietary fiber is that portion of plant-based foods (such as fruits, legumes, vegetables, and whole grains) that cannot be completely digested. Scientists maintain that high-fiber diets reduce cholesterol levels and cancer rates.

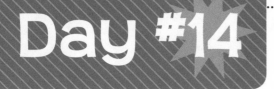

Day #14

Marshall: I want my body to be able to run. I have said that before and it keeps coming back to me. It's my gauge I guess. You always need a goal; it's the key to success. I look at kids at school, on the playground, and they can zip and dash. I am always being chased, and I don't like that because I always get caught.

spaghetti squash

Spaghetti squash is an awesome side dish for a busy household. It is available all year long and can be stored at room temperature for many weeks. This makes it a super-easy ingredient to have on hand. We bake ours whole, let them cool, and then cut them in half and scoop out the seeds (just like you do for a pumpkin). Take a fork and gently slide it over the pulp toward you, and it will come up like spaghetti noodles. We love ours tossed with basic olive oil, garlic, salt, and pepper. But you can even add some yummy spaghetti sauce from a jar. Spaghetti squash is very versatile for a low-calorie dish packed full of nutrients, and it doesn't have the heavy squash taste so many people oppose.

Alex: The passing of an item from generation to generation within a family creates an heirloom. I come across heirloom items daily in my antiques business. But now that we have started PSM, it has become more apparent to me that habits and feelings can be heirlooms as well. What do I want my children to cherish and hold dear to them? What heirlooms and traditions will they hand down to the next generation? I will have to explore this further within myself and make a conscientious effort to recognize those things that could become important heirlooms.

I'm starting to feel really good. My shorts are more comfortable. I have so much more energy. My mom tries hard to do things with me, but she has a schedule. So I try to do things on my own, like riding my bike or working on this Army bunker I'm making in the yard. It's a big hole I have dug, and I move scrap wood and firewood around it for defenses.

For exercise, play a follow-the-leader game. You can do this anywhere at any time: out in the yard, at a park, or even in the house. But you change leaders each day. One day the child leads and he or she gets to choose anything involving movement: skipping, hopping over a chair, or balancing on a log, for example. The next day, someone else leads, doing leapfrogs, passing by the radio and turning it on to dance to a song, and then moving on. Do it for a set time limit and make a rule that the followers cannot argue with what is chosen. Remind them that they get to lead soon and can add all kinds of cruel payback as punishment.

Six Benefits of Regular Physical Activity

1. Exercise improves your mood. Need to blow off some steam after a stressful day? A workout at the gym or a brisk thirty-minute walk can help you calm down.

2. Exercise combats chronic diseases. Worried about heart disease? Hoping to prevent osteoporosis? Physical activity might be the ticket.

3. Exercise helps you manage your weight. Want to drop those excess pounds? Trade some couch time for walking or other physical activities.

4. Exercise boosts your energy level. Winded by grocery shopping or household chores? Don't throw in the towel. Regular physical activity can leave you breathing easier.

5. Exercise promotes better sleep. Struggling to fall asleep? Or stay asleep? It might help to boost your physical activity during the day.

6. Exercise can be—gasp—fun! Wondering what to do on a Saturday afternoon? Looking for an activity that suits the entire family? Get physical!

Noodles with Ham and Tomatoes

This is one of those quick meals that we just threw together, but it ended up being really delicious and healthy. We had diced ham in the freezer and a bunch of garden tomatoes to use. We combined the ham and chopped tomatoes with a little garlic, olive oil, and basil. We sautéed the mixture for a few minutes, placed it over whole-wheat noodles, and then violà: dinner!

Marshall and Jordan show off their noodles.

Overcooked, mushy noodles don't do anything but create a texture like gelatinous goo in your mouth. The term *al dente* literally means "to the tooth." That means that the noodle doesn't squish between your teeth when you bite into it, but rather has a firm texture. It shouldn't be hard and crunchy, though. It is a very fine line in between. Healthy carbs are important for exercise energy, so investigate the best ways to make your whole-grain pasta *al dente*.

Marshall walks hard here and explains how our videos are created.

Day 14
Video 2

Track

Helpful Hint!

Here's an idea to help your kids curb the desire to eat out at unhealthy restaurants. Buy a piggy bank and tell yourself and your kids that every time you wanted to or were about to eat at someplace unhealthy, you instead put the money that it would have cost in the piggy bank. After a period of time—say, six months—the kids get what is in the piggy bank. Or maybe you split the money!

Your Journey!

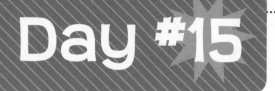

Day #15

Marshall: The reason why bullies always pick on you is because they are insecure. When I say insecure I mean they are feeling bad, they are mad about something. Hopefully they will grow out of it. There are a lot reasons why bullies pick on you. The main reason is the fact a lot of the time they are just upset about something that has to do with them. If they are larger and so are you, chances are that they want to pick on you to feel better about themselves. A good solution to keeping people from bullying you is to simply ignore them. That doesn't mean tell them to leave you alone. I mean pretend that they are not even there. That they don't even exist. Tell yourself "he's not there" and then focus on something that makes you feel good.

Simple Guacamole

To me, the two keys to good guacamole are to keep the ingredients minimal and not pulverize the avocado. I use a butter knife to slice through the avocado in the bowl and dice it instead of mashing it with a fork. Then I use a large spoon to fold all the ingredients together without mashing the tender avocado any more than is needed. Basically, I don't care for guacamole paste.

- » 3 avocados
- » ½ lemon
- » Splash of Worcestershire sauce
- » Lots of garlic
- » Pepper (no salt is needed because it's already on the chips)
- » Couple spoonfuls of fresh homemade salsa or high-quality jarred salsa
- » Tortilla chips

Mix all the ingredients together, chill, and serve with tortilla chips.

Take a look at what an actual portion size of tortilla chips looks like so you don't overeat.

Alex: Here we are at day fifteen, and there are moments when I am even more willing and wanting to continue with this lifelong change. I feel energized and in control, proud and ambitious of other things I can tackle. But there are equally as many moments that I am feeling like it would be so much easier to return to previous habits, to not have to put so much work into it. You know that period in the day when you just want to take a nap and imagine things would continue on their path without your involvement. You would wake up and step right into the movement, as if not even missing a beat, and continue as if the nap had never occurred. I suppose Marshall is probably feeling the same way.

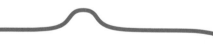

Milk and juice are my favorite, but I am trying to choose more water over other things. Sometimes I even make flavored water just so it's not so boring by adding fresh squeezed lemon or orange juice. It makes sense; your body is mostly made out of water, so you need to replace it. Your body is not made out of milk, even though milk helps your bones and teeth. This is going to be hard for me 'cause I really do like milk.

If your family members are big milk drinkers like mine, be aware that even the calories in 2 percent milk (which is the leanest I can stand) can add up. We used to throw the whole gallon on the table during meals for convenient refills. No more. Now it's one glass and then water!

Who is Louis Pasteur?

Milk, a natural drink, is one of our most nutritionally complete foods, adding protein, fat, minerals, and vitamins to your diet.

However, milk contains bacteria that—when improperly handled—may create unsafe conditions. Most of the bacteria in fresh milk are either harmless or beneficial. But changes in the health of an animal or the milk handler or contaminants from polluted water, dirt, manure, vermin, air, etc., can make raw milk potentially dangerous.

Louis Pasteur developed pasteurization, which is a moderate but exact heat treatment of milk. Pasteurization kills bacteria that produce disease and delays spoilage in milk.

French Dip

Day 15 Video 2

» 1 large beef chuck roast (trim any fat off)
» 4 cups beef broth
» 1 sprig rosemary
» Lots of garlic
» 1 onion, chopped
» Lots of fresh mushrooms, sliced
» 1 bay leaf
» 1 poblano pepper, sliced

Place the roast in a slow cooker or roast pan. Add all ingredients.

Cover and cook on high for 5 to 6 hours in the slow cooker, or bake at 350°F in the roast pan, until beef is tender, probably about 2½ hrs.

Remove the meat from the broth mixture and shred it with a fork.

Serve the beef in a whole-wheat hoagie bun, and spoon the mushrooms, onions, and peppers over top of the sandwiches. Poor the broth into small cups, and dip the sandwiches in it.

Marshall puts the slow-cooker recipe together here.

Avocados are jokingly known as alligator pears due to the bumps on their skin. There are approximately five hundred variations of avocado, but I have always classified them in two types: California avocados and Florida avocados. California avocados are smaller and darker skinned, while the Florida ones are larger and bright green.

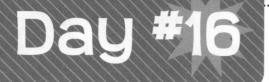

Day #16

Marshall: *I think it's unfair that some kids got a chance that I have not had. Everyone else was born skinny and I was born fat. This didn't just happen to me last year; I've been dealing with it my entire life. I think that people who are born big like me are more sensitive to things, and it's gonna be harder for us. But that's our life. In a way, I am glad it has happened to me because I will overcome it and I will be stronger.*

Alex: I hope you have noticed that we have worked very hard in sharing our information with you while also doing our best not to lead you down a road of musts. Practice moderation. Avoid extremes. Those are our only musts. We have, however, tried to provide you with commonly agreed-upon information and facts so that you may make your own decisions.

We've tried to bring an awareness of natural, organic, and gluten-free food into our Portion Size Me program. We personally don't seek out items with those terms, but they are becoming more and more prevalent—not only at specialty stores, but also at regular grocery stores—so we wanted to make sure we acknowledge them. If you set a goal to eat an all organic or vegan diet, more power to you; you're braver than I am.

We provide here definitions from the U.S. federal government for reference only because the government is the entity that approves a label on a product. It should be noted that there are many self-governing agencies that provide terms and definitions that wholesalers, producers, and suppliers do cooperatively adhere to.

Polenta

Polenta is a corn-based product, and I have always seen it in the stores in tubes in the produce section. So I looked into the ingredients, and then I looked up a recipe and tried grilling it. I have experimented several times with cutting it into different thicknesses to get a crispier versus meatier texture. I also really love the fresh tomato, basil, and mozzarella salad, and here I have mixed the two with success, in my opinion. And because of the heaviness of the corn, this meal fills you up beyond what you would expect from a lighter salad so it can be a full meal instead of a side.

- » 1 package polenta, sliced thin and either grilled or baked until crispy
- » Fresh tomatoes, quartered
- » Fresh basil, gently torn into pieces
- » Part skim mozzarella, cut into thin slices
- » Olive oil
- » Balsamic vinegar
- » Salt and pepper
- » Crushed red pepper, like the kind found at pizza parlors (optional)

Place a few polenta crisps on individual plates.

In a bowl, gently mix the tomatoes, basil, and mozzarella in oil and vinegar. You be the judge of the amount of ingredients. I like basil, so I go heavy on the basil. I also like the vinegar, so I go heavier on that too. Marshall likes a little less vinegar. However, don't drown the ingredients: you just want the oil and vinegar tastes to be subtle.

Lightly add salt and pepper to taste, and add crushed red pepper for a little bite, if you'd like.

Spoon the salad mixture over half of the polenta lying on the plates. If you leave half of the polenta uncovered, you can still get to enjoy bites with good texture and not have all of the polenta absorbing the oil and vinegar from the salad.

I read that 1 pound of body fat is equal to 3,500 calories. I believe that it is generally agreed that muscle weighs more than fat. What does all that mean to me, and what am I going to tell Marshall? Forget the scale. It's a tool, but it is not what is going to assist in long-term behavior change. In fact, I might be so bold to say that it could derail long-term behavior change. For example, what if you start working out and start building more muscle? You may still be burning calories and fat, but the scale may not reflect that.

The use of terminology on food packages can have a big impact and sway our decisions to purchase a product. One such term is "organic." This gets confusing, but since we are asking you to read labels, you may have seen the USDA certified organic seal on some products. The National Organic Program is a marketing arm housed within the USDA. Their goal is to provide consistent standards for the companies that want to put that seal on their packaging. Once a product is certified by a third-party inspector, you can be assured that it is at least 95% organic.

snack suggestions

Day 16
Video 1

Snacking is a necessity, but it's important to choose the right snack. It's also key to make sure you're snacking for the right reasons—for example, because you're hungry, not because you're tired or bored. Snacks that fill you up with some fiber or mostly water will keep you feeling full and hydrated until the next time you eat. Snacking on a candy bar or chips satisfies your sweet or salty craving but can leave you feeling hungry a short while later. But you can satisfy those little devils by enhancing a healthy snack. Take a piece of watermelon for example. Want to make it sweeter? Then add a touch of honey or agave nectar. Craving salt? Sprinkle a little salt on the juicy melon. What if you are the sweet and sour type? Squeeze a lime over your slice of watermelon.

Watch Marshall put together a *Portion Size Me*–approved snack.

How your taste buds react to food can be described as five basic tastes: sweet, sour, salty, bitter, and *umami*. The latter is the Japanese word for "savory." Think about those five tastes and how we altered them with our watermelon slices.

Day #17

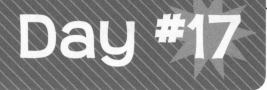

Marshall: What is "making it?" Well I am making it right now. I was not happy, so now I am changing. There are so many good things happening, and PSM is part of it. I feel good. I'm happy! I'm not just waking up and getting through each day...I'm actually enjoying my days! I know I am going to feel good if I make a few small changes and keep up with them. That's making it for right now. I just have to keep up with all this, and then that is really making it! You see, it doesn't really matter to me if you are 1,000 pounds or 11 pounds, as long as you are happy. But I was not happy, so now I am changing.

Alex: What does a mom bring to the table? Your plate. A story. Ritual. Sanctity. Comfort. Free therapy. Compassion. Understanding. Laughter. Insight. Support. That is a mom's easy investment in the future.

Warm Salad

This is really onion soup, but we add so many delicious goodies that it becomes a warm and satisfying salad. Don't be afraid to try this just because you don't care for onions. That particular pungent taste cooks out into a wonderful broth. You can cut these onions up thinly by hand, but it's worth the investment of a mandolin slicer to do this for you.

- » 2 tablespoons butter
- » 6 onions, sliced as thinly as possible
- » Lots of fresh garlic
- » 8 to 10 cups chicken or beef broth
- » Pepper
- » Low-fat mozzarella cheese, shredded
- » Bacon, microwaved until crispy and then chopped
- » Tomatoes, diced
- » Cilantro, chopped
- » Scallions, chopped
- » Croutons (refer to Dinner Day 9 for recipe)
- » Avocado, diced
- » Water chestnuts, diced

Melt the butter in a large stockpot and add the onions and garlic. Cook the onions and garlic until they are almost transparent, about 15 minutes. Add the broth and simmer for about 20 to 30 minutes. Add pepper to taste (there should be plenty of salt from the broth).

Now here is the salad part. Fill 8 separate bowls with the mozzarella, bacon, tomatoes, cilantro, scallions, croutons, avocado, and water chestnuts, and set them up buffet style. Serve the soup super hot and allow your family or guests to fill up on all the delectable toppings as they would like.

Serve up some fun and serve your food in a sundae glass. Why not? It's smaller than a regular bowl or plate, and you will automatically feel like you're eating a special treat.

Day 17
Video 1

Here are my tips for peeling onions. As goofy as this sounds, wear swimming goggles. You will thank me. Or you can set up a fan to blow the onion fumes away from your face. **See my tip in action.**

Onions, Oh My!

A member of the lily family, the onion is flavorful and aromatic when cooked or pungent and sharp when eaten raw. There are many varieties, but the kinds typically found in the grocery store are red, white, and yellow onions, plus some special sweet onions like Vidalia and Walla Walla. The latter are named for the locations in which they are grown. When their skins are thicker, they are considered winter onions and have a longer storage life; summer onions have thinner skins and a relatively short shelf life. Leeks and green onions, which are also known as scallions, are smaller. They have long green stalks attached, which are edible.

George Washington used to eat a cooked onion whenever he was beginning to feel ill. His homeopathic remedy probably assisted in his recovery, as onions are packed full of vitamins. But folks usually shy away from onions because they can sting your eyes when you chop them. When sliced, the onion releases sulfur, which was absorbed from the earth as it grew. This gas mixes with the natural lubricants of your eyes and turns into sulfuric acid. Ouch! Your eyes tear naturally to try to flush the irritant out, and rubbing your eyes, also a natural reaction, may actually make the situation worse.

Bread Pudding

Chef Paul Prudhomme is one of my favorite chefs, and I make his bread pudding every Thanksgiving. I hope he doesn't mind that I changed things here to be able to make it more frequently, but he should rest assured that I will stick with his original recipe for my Thanksgiving holiday.

- » ½ cup sugar
- » ½ cup brown sugar
- » 2 (12-ounce) cans light evaporated milk
- » 3 eggs
- » 1 teaspoon vanilla extract
- » 1 teaspoon cinnamon
- » 1 teaspoon nutmeg
- » ½ teaspoon salt
- » ¼ teaspoon cream of tartar
- » ¼ teaspoon ground ginger
- » 4 slices white bread, toasted (feel free to use the ends of the loaf or stale pieces; they make for the best bread pudding)
- » 4 slices whole-wheat bread, toasted (again, feel free to use the loaf ends or stale slices)

Add the sugar, evaporated milk, eggs, vanilla extract, cinnamon, nutmeg, salt, cream of tartar, and ginger to a large mixing bowl and mix well. You may use an electric mixer for this if you wish.

Tear the toasted bread slices into small pieces and add them to milk mixture, pushing down on the sides of the bowl with a rubber spatula until the bread has absorbed as much of the mixture as it can.

Place the mixture in an ungreased baking dish and bake at 450°F degrees for about 25 minutes or until browned. Cool and serve.

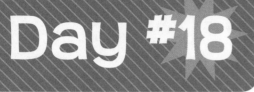

Day #18

Grilled Chicken Tenders

I just wanted to remind you that zesty Italian salad dressing (now available in a high-fructose corn syrup free version) is a great marinade for meats and vegetables. It's simple and quick and really brings out the natural flavors of the items you are marinating. Plan on picking a bottle of it up the next time you are at the grocery store so that you'll have it on hand.

What we like to do is throw everything together in a big bowl to marinate. Fresh, raw, un-breaded chicken tenders, asparagus, mushrooms, corn on the cob, Brussels sprouts, onions, lots of garlic cloves. Anything you have on hand. This is a great opportunity to use any frozen vegetables you may have. One thing we add, but it is of course your choice, is a splash of hot sauce. My preference is the Chinese Sriracha sauce. Let it all sit in the refrigerator, covered, marinating for the whole day. Then just throw it all on the grill or griddle when you're ready to eat. You could even put it on a baking sheet and put it under the broiler if you wish. Make sure you cook the chicken thoroughly. The point is to anticipate when you have a busy schedule and use an easily available, uncomplicated marinade to make a quick and healthy meal.

Watch Marshall easily put together a chicken tender dinner.

Marshall: If you live in a rural area like I do, there probably isn't much stuff to do. There probably aren't very many kids to play with, and there probably isn't a lot of concrete around for you to skateboard or ride your bike on. So you really need to keep on your parents to help you get out. Like me and my mom right now are trying to go to the tennis courts almost every day. Pick something you like and then it will be easier to do it more often. Sometimes we ride our bikes, other times we hit tennis balls, and then there is a baseball field we run around. And that's really it!

Alex: As you can see, this project has been a great opportunity to step back and reevaluate the balance in our lives between family, self, and work. I would imagine Marshall feels a similar sense of change other than just how his body is feeling. He may not be able to articulate it, but I am sure he feels the additional peace, happiness, and comfort this period has brought to our household.

> Before PSM I was eating faster and I wouldn't think about what I was tasting. I wouldn't think about what the food tasted like. I would just scarf it down. Nowadays I eat a lot slower. I don't just scarf everything down. I eat and taste the food as if every bite was the last bite I would ever have. I have to make myself slow down, so now I appreciate food a lot more than I did before.

I have started talking to Marshall about his tummy's needs. I made it a bit more complicated than needed, though, so a friend made a brilliant suggestion: a full meter. So now I ask Marshall where his full meter is. We discuss it in percentages, or you could just describe it on a scale from one to ten, with ten being full. I am also trying to reassure him that 80 percent full is OK, and that he can probably get to the next meal or snack time without eating any more.

The grilled cheese sandwich has been around since the 1920s, when bread was inexpensive and processed cheeses became readily available. Nobody knows who exactly created this simple and endearing concoction, but children will no doubt continue to enjoy this timeless tradition for generations to come.

Grilled Cheese

You're probably thinking, "Really, I don't need to buy a book to teach me how to make grilled cheese." True, you don't. But I wanted to include this recipe because every kid knows what grilled cheese is, and now we can teach them to make it a bit healthier. And you never know: if your kid knows how to make himself grilled cheese and some pasta and pesto, he may not be living at home with you at age twenty-seven. If you have not been able to switch completely to whole-grain bread, here is an opportunity to use one slice of whole grain and once slice of your favorite. Instead of spreading butter on the outside of the bread to make it crispy, brush on a little olive oil. Choose lower fat cheese and consider adding a slice or two of tomato. I even add a slice of yellow onion.

Throw away any meat that has been at room temperature for two hours or more. When in doubt, throw it out!

Mom's Quick Tip!
A hearty meal is influenced as much by its appearance as it is by feeling full and satisfied. We tend to not think our meal is complete until we have emptied our plates, and the larger the plate, the larger our meal. Put your large beautiful plates away for special occasions and use smaller ones for daily use. It's a simple trick to the eye and to your health. Little kids love little packages too. Many dollar stores sell custard cups and little sauce cups. Try serving meals in two or three of these little cups or bowls and place them on a plate. It's just plain fun for them; it makes them feel special; and, best of all, it's portion sized.

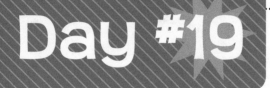

Marshall: I really like my veggies steamed or roasted; they have a lot more flavor like that. I like a little resistance when I bite them. I like that bit of crunch. I don't like to bite into mush. Stewed and roasted veggies bring out a little more elegant flavor. I like adding new veggies, but I also miss the traditional meals we used to have, though I know that's not fair to ourselves to continue doing that. I mean the bad way we used to make vegetables, like covering them in butter and cheese. I miss that, but ya know, it's Ok. I like the new way we are making them. I didn't really realize vegetables had so many flavors by themselves.

Scallop Kabobs

Throw some fresh or thawed frozen scallops in a large mixing bowl with some whole cloves of garlic and cherry tomatoes. Toss in some light, zesty Italian salad dressing, and marinate the scallops for about an hour. Soak wooden skewers in water while you're marinating, as this will prevent the skewers from burning.

Gently skewer all the ingredients in any fun combination you want, and place the skewers on a hot grill.

The scallops and tomatoes are very fragile and do not take long at all to cook, maybe 2 minutes on each side. Use a spatula to turn the skewers, as the scallops may stick to the grill and tear.

We just gobble these up, but you can serve them over rice or couscous if you'd like.

Watch Marshall prepare scallop kabobs.

Alex: I used to make nutritious, colorful, and delightful meals all the time. But someone inevitably complained or moaned or argued about eating it. Often everyone complained about different things. They said thank you in their own ungrateful ways, like: "The meat was fine, but everything else was gross." After years, I really did just give up. I'm being honest. It's not that hard to be appreciative and grateful. Or at least thankful. How does the adage go... "There are starving people somewhere, so be grateful you have something on your plate."

We also had a disagreement in our family, among the adults, about how to teach the children how to appreciate what they have in front of them. One of us was happy if they "did a good job" and at least tried everything. The other was the clean-the-plate person. I don't believe we really ever resolved that parental difference; we just sidestepped it until the kids outgrew that stage or we finally gave up. But that time period stands as a record in the foundation of the kids' lives.

I bring all this negative baggage to you in the hopes that if you have similar issues in your home, you address them now and not let them become a permanent pattern. I want to inspire you to keep cooking and providing for your family. Although mealtimes can be frustrating when you have young children who are picky eaters, it really is a short time in the grand scheme of things.

Look what I did for some exercise today, a homemade slip 'n' slide.

Try planning and eating some meals with your fingers, such as the scallop kabobs. It gives you different sensations and takes you a little longer to eat. We mostly use utensils and cut our food into safe, bite-size pieces. But feeling the food, its texture or firmness, and having to tear pieces to the right size—basically playing with your food and ignoring all proper table manners—can be a fun way to slow down and make more of a connection with what you are putting in your mouth. If that seems gross to you, remember that many cultures in the Middle East eat exclusively with their fingers.

What's in Your Seafood?

Mock (imitation) seafood has been around in Asian cultures for a very long time. And now many countries make use of readily available, "undesirable" fish to replace the more expensive varieties that are becoming scarcer, such as crab and lobster. This fodder fish is minced and then rinsed to remove its odor. Then it is pulverized and mixed with other products, like starch and MSG, until it is the desired consistency. Next it is seasoned, shaped, and packaged. Often you cannot tell the difference in flavor between mock and real seafood. Sometimes, texture and shape can be a clue. Even fish sold at a restaurant can be replaced with its more common and less desirable mate. For example, a famed Florida grouper sandwich can really be made with tilapia.

crab cakes

I grew up just outside San Francisco, and I remember throwing out a crab trap on my way to school, then picking up the Dungeness crab on my way home. We boiled it in a crab boil and picked at it for the rest of the evening. But I do not recall ever making crab cakes. So here we go! This is perfect for special occasions.

» 1 pound lump or fresh crab meat, drained of all liquids
» 2 egg whites
» 3 tablespoons light mayo
» Dash Worcestershire sauce
» A dozen crushed whole-wheat crackers, or the equivalent amount of whole-wheat bread crumbs or Panko crumbs
» Salt and pepper
» A bit of garlic (This is the only time we advise using a small amount of garlic.)
» A few scallions, minced
» A couple pinches of Old Bay seasoning, if you have it
» Lots of fresh lemon juice

In a large bowl, gently but thoroughly combine all the ingredients except the lemon, and use your hands to form four patties. If the mixture is too dry to form patties, add a bit more lemon juice. If the mixture is too wet, add more crumbs.

Coat a skillet with cooking spray and warm it over medium heat. Add the crab cakes and cook 10 minutes on each side, or until crispy. Squeeze lemon juice over the cakes just before serving.

Frankly, scallop, I don't give a clam!

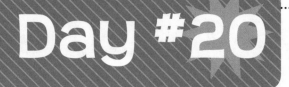

Day #20

Marshall: Genetics are holding me back, but they are not the excuse. If I make excuses, I won't make it. I think genetics are probably about 88 percent of the reason that I am this big. I feel like I don't have enough friends encouraging me. I feel like my family is doing 100 percent to help me, but I could use some support from my friends too. I know my family will always be there. But my friends think of me and say wow, he could be a great kid one day; he just needs to lose weight. I don't care about myself and how I am, but I know everyone else really cares for me, and they want me to have a better life than what I am starting out as.

I don't care for myself because I am this way, but I want to feel good about myself.

Alex: Other cultures around the world eat a large variety of food, yet they don't have the same level of health problems that our nation does. Some cultures eat mostly meat, some eat only veggies and grains, some eat rotten blubber, and others eat tons of white rice. We even have a government that has stepped in to try to outline its best recommendations to keep us on the right track. When I think about why this might be, what really makes our dietary habits different from other cultures', two things keep coming to mind: We must just be eating too much! And we are not eating enough real food that our bodies know what to do with. I'm aware that there are many other factors involved, but quantity and quality are two giant factors I can easily control, and we can have success within our family with Portion Size Me.

Ethiopian Bread

Marshall asked to make some real bread, and that brought up memories of making bread as a kid, baby-sitting my dough next to the water heater. Marshall and I tried this bread from Ethiopia. This does have a lot of butter in it, so make it a side dish for something like kabobs.

- » 1 packet dry active yeast (make sure it's fresh)
- » ¼ cup lukewarm water
- » 1 egg, beaten
- » ½ cup honey
- » 1 teaspoon ground coriander
- » 1 teaspoon ground cinnamon
- » ½ teaspoon ground cloves
- » 1 teaspoon salt
- » 1 cup milk, warmed
- » 6 tablespoons butter, melted
- » 4½ cups whole-wheat flour

In a small bowl, stir together the yeast and warm water. Set for about 10 minutes.

In a large bowl, beat together the egg, honey, spices, and salt until smooth. Stir in the milk and melted butter. Then add the yeast and water mixture.

Stir in the flour, ½ cup at a time, mixing to form a soft, smooth dough. Do not add all of the flour if the dough gets too stiff. Add more flour if the dough is too sticky.

Move the dough to a lightly floured work surface and knead for about 10 minutes to form a smooth, elastic dough.

Place the dough in a large, lightly oiled bowl, cover it with plastic wrap, and let the dough rise in a warm place until doubled in size, about 1½ hours.

Move the dough again to a lightly floured work surface. Punch it down and knead it for about 1 minute. Form the dough into a round and place it on an oiled baking sheet. Allow it to rise again for another 30 to 45 minutes.

Preheat the oven to 325°F. Place the bread on a baking sheet in the oven and bake 45 minutes to 1 hour, or until bread is lightly browned and sounds hollow when you tap on it. Remove and cool the bread slightly before slicing.

Our goal is to walk and exercise thirty minutes a day. Yesterday we did twenty-two minutes. So, yea! We will get there.

Are you supposed to wash your meat before you cook it? I never have because I figured that anything naughty on the surface would be eliminated when the meat is cooked sufficiently. But Marshall asked, so I decided to look into it. Apparently, there is quite an extreme disparity of thoughts on this. Many believe you should wash meat before cooking it, while others seem to believe that doing so may spread *E. coli* around your sink and work area and cause future contamination. This is something to think about as you make your own decisions and introduce your kids to the kitchen.

With over five hundred varieties of pasta and its popularity across so many lands, this food is a versatile staple to have in the pantry. In many North African countries, couscous, ground semolina, is a staple. It is smaller than rice grains and adds a wonderful texture to any dish.

Garbage Bobs

We are making another skewered dish because we had so much fun with the scallops yesterday. You can use any meat you have left in the freezer and all the wonderful veggies and fruits you can think of. Try bell peppers, mushrooms, yellow squash, zucchini, eggplant, tomatoes, onions, and pineapple. If you don't have time to marinate the ingredients, that's OK; just season with salt, pepper, and lots of garlic powder. Cut everything into chunks, skewer the pieces, and throw the kabobs on the grill. Kids can do all the prepping for this meal, and best of all: no dishes! OK, maybe you'll have one pot, because couscous goes great with the garbage bobs.

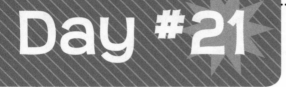

Day #21

Marshall: We have to complete a mile every year for the school fitness test. Well, I am tired of being the last one done. I don't wanna have to sit there and say, "Yea, I'm the last one. So what? I don't care." I do care! I want to be first! But I can't right now with my body as it is. I just try my best, but it's not even close to other kids. Once I started PSM, I could run faster. Once I pick it up a little more, it will be a lot easier for me to run because my body will be in better shape.

Alex: You are the product of your environment, I believe. But I do also believe you can change your environment.

For example, some families are into sports. In our family, Dan plays hockey with the boys a couple nights a week, Jordan swims on the local club team, Marshall plays baseball and basketball, and I play tennis. Whenever the TV is left on for background noise, it's tuned to ESPN. The entire household is constantly moving from events to meets to training. They have an athletic environment that they are all products of.

Imagine all the possible environments that exist, how they influence us, and how you may be able to change your own environment. For example, my husband likes to read, but in our household, he doesn't get any quiet time to do so. So he changed his environment by waking up an hour earlier, before the rest of the family wakes up, to fit in his much-needed intellectual time. Adding a family game night can change your environment, at least for one night. Setting a day on the weekend to go explore a park trail, river, lake, or waterfall, can begin to change your family's environment to a more exploratory and outdoorsy one.

Kids can change their environment too, but they just need some guidance to help them discover how to do it. Do they want to make more friends? They can join the local YMCA or a 4-H club. Do they want to learn a new hobby? You can sign them up for a class. My point is that you have the choice to lead and create your environment.

Bulgogi

» Flank steak or top sirloin, cut into thin slices
» ¼ cup soy sauce
» 1 tablespoon sugar or brown sugar
» 1 tablespoon sesame oil
» 1 tablespoon sesame seeds
» Lots of garlic, minced
» Salt and pepper
» Bunch scallions, sliced thin

Mix all the ingredients in a large bowl. Cover and marinate for at least 2 hours. (Overnight in the fridge would be the best.)

Cook the mixture either on an outdoor grill on top of aluminum foil or under your oven's broiler until the meat is thoroughly cooked, about six minutes on each side. Serve with lots of fresh veggies and over brown rice if you wish.

Watch Marshall discuss the importance of staying hydrated.

Day 21
Video 1

I want to get this stomach off me, and I want to lose weight from my thighs. If you have smaller thighs, you can bring your legs up higher. I want to get the muscles better so I can run for longer periods. If I can work on my cardiovascular health, I can run longer distances without being winded so much.

One neat thing about organized sports play is the rarely mentioned benefit of motivation and commitment. I don't mean commitment to coaches or team members, but instead to a group of people who are waiting for you at a designated time. That by itself is motivating, even outside of the sports play.

How can we replicate that outside sense of commitment in the absence of participating in activities? Here are a couple of ideas. Many communities have animal shelters that need volunteers. Go walk a dog a couple of times a week. Clean some pens or participate in a fund-raising or adoption event. If you're an animal person, maybe if you feel that the animals need you, it will help motivate you. Or why not try starting a community garden? Those plants need you!

We all know that our bodies are mostly made of water. The foods we choose to eat can help keep us hydrated too. Melons, oranges, iceberg lettuce, and tomatoes are just some fruits and vegetables that contain a lot of water in them naturally. If you are out in the heat or are exercising, it's important to not only replace what you lose but also to keep up with regular hydration.

The American College of Sports Medicine (ACSM) defines aerobic exercise as "any activity that uses large muscle groups, can be maintained continuously, and is rhythmic in nature." It is a type of exercise that overloads the heart and lungs and causes them to work harder than they do at rest. The important idea behind aerobic exercise today is to get up and get moving! There are more activities than ever to choose from, whether it is a new activity or an old one. Find something you enjoy doing that keeps your heart rate elevated for a continuous time period, and get moving to a healthier life. —Georgia State University department of kinesiology and health

Track

Helpful Hint!
Your body is your currency. If you invest in your health by being physically active, you get to do more things and you pay less in healthcare bills.

Your Journey!

Have you ever noticed the logo of Shell Oil at local gas stations? Well, that shell is actually a scallop shell, and it is one of the most recognized shell shapes. A scallop is an edible bivalve, like an oyster. There are larger sea scallops and smaller bay scallops, and both have a delicate, sweet taste. Sometimes scallops are faked by using shark fin.

Track

Your Journey!

Do you have any favorite family recipes? Something your grandmother used to make? Jot it down here so you remember to share it with your children and teach them how to make it.

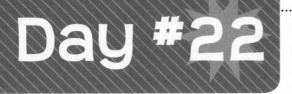

Day #22

Marshall: We always have a party at Christmastime, and we have this green foam tower my mom got from a florist friend. We use toothpicks and attach cherry tomatoes, olives, and cheese cubes shaped like stars all over it to put on our buffet. We've done it for several years and people think it's really cute on the table. You see, it's fun to play with food. You get good food and creativity. Why not give it a try? It doesn't have to be a holiday.

Alex: It takes time to change your family's behaviors. Just think about changing a single personal behavior. It could be a big one like smoking or a smaller one like picking up your clothes from the floor. Now imagine changing multiple behaviors from multiple people. I can see that the issues we are addressing here (laziness, boredom, portion sizes, mindfulness, etc.) are like an onion, and we have to peel away each layer and change individual behaviors one at a time before we can get to the next layer. And I would anticipate that we may have to readdress behaviors several times. That's OK—we will take this slow and steady like the tortoise and not bounce around like the hare.

sour cream dip for fruit

- » 1 tablespoon honey, agave nectar, or stevia (a natural herb)
- » ½ cup low-fat sour cream

Mix the ingredients together and serve chilled. Use as a dip for your favorite cut-up fruit.

I have started filling up on the healthy stuff first at meals. I like eating all my veggies on my plate before anything else. I think it's a good choice.

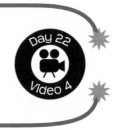

Day 22
Video 4

» Challenge yourself to take your favorite restaurant meal and make it healthier.

Fungus Among Us!

Fungi are used primarily for culinary, medicinal, and psychoactive purposes. There are hundreds, if not thousands, of mushroom strains that are eaten by people around the world: shiitake, oyster, truffle, wood ear, and button mushrooms are commonplace fungi that are cooked or eaten raw. Fungi also play a key role in traditional medicine, including Chinese and Japanese holistic medicine. The reishi or lingzhi mushroom, for example, is widely recognized for boosting the immune system. Certain mushrooms are consumed for their psychoactive properties. They were consumed as early as 1,000 BCE, when cultures in Mexico and Guatemala worshipped mushroom gods and built temples and carved mushroom statues in honor of them. But remember, never pick and eat a wild mushroom.

Portobello Mushroom Burgers

Day 22
Videos 1-3

When it comes to a typical burger, we find the bun to be the real culprit. Perhaps you are one of the disciplined humanoids who can go bun free or eat it as an open-face burger and thereby only eat half the bun. We are not. A friend handed us a book called *Eat This, Not That* by David Zinczenko, and while reading it, Marshall discovered that a portobello mushroom burger popular in a major chain restaurant is actually quite horrible for you. So he decided to make a healthy version, by replacing the bun with the mushroom.

Watch Marshall create his portobello mushroom burgers.

Many states require a sanitation health rating for restaurants. "Sanitation" may be defined in this case as "safety from contamination." Just like at home, the temperatures that foods are cooked to and stored at, along with chef and workspace cleanliness, are extremely important at restaurants. Oftentimes, due to large numbers of employees and the quantity of foods moving through the kitchen, it can be harder to keep sanitation levels up to the required standards in restaurants. Next time you are out, look to see if your chosen restaurant prominently displays a health rating, and look around to notice its cleanliness.

This mushroom walks into a birthday party. The birthday boy says, "Hey, you can't be in here." And the mushroom says, "Why not? I'm a fungi!"

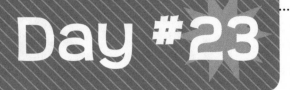

Day #23

Marshall: I am extremely lucky that I got the opportunity to have such an excellent mother. My mom is one in a billion. Ha! I guess I got lucky. She is so nice to me and actually helps me to care about how I turn out when I grow up. That she actually, you know, cares is really important to me. Most kids around me have parents that are way too protective or don't appreciate their maturity. My mom, well, she is just realistic. She will tell me I am not making a good decision or stuff like that. If she told me what to do and what to eat, and if she only let me watch one hour of TV a day, she would be helping me in my childhood, but she would also be making it harder in my adulthood. How would I know how to do things as an adult if I don't have decisions to learn from now? Right now I think I have a good balance with my mom between the things she teaches me and the times I want to tell her to get off my back and leave me alone.

Stuffed London Broil

Day 23 Video 1

"London broil" is not a cut of steak but rather a generic term for marinating, cooking, and cutting against the grain of a lean piece of meat. Traditionally, flank steak was used, but over time, other cuts of meat have become used for London broil.

We marinate ours in equal amounts of soy sauce and balsamic vinegar, with a couple dashes of salt, pepper, and ginger. Then we cut small slits (maybe 15 or 20 total) randomly on both sides of the steak and push a small garlic clove into each slit.

We either cook it on the grill or under the broiler in the oven. Sometimes you lose a garlic clove or two on the grill, but that's OK.

Next, we cut the steak as thinly as possible on the bias (cutting the meat at a 45-degree angle), and serve. Delightful.

Watch Marshall create his marinade for London broil.

Alex: I don't want to get into a whole parenting conversation here, but I do want to share that I typically choose to educate rather than dictate as a strategy with my children. Now, I know many of you are thinking that children are young and do not have the maturity to multi-task, to be safe, quick, and skillful in the kitchen and need to just be told what to do. There is validity to that. Unfortunately that does not come naturally to me, and I see the want and hunger to learn and be independent in their little hazel eyes. That doesn't mean that I don't sometimes say "because I said so" to end an argument or say "do exactly as I tell you." But as an example, I would prefer to work with Marshall in the kitchen and teach him about cooking and controlling his portions rather than serve him his meal and put a lock on the pantry doors. What's the old proverb? You can give a man a fish and feed him for a day, or you can teach a man to fish and feed him for life. Something like that!

> This is feeling really good. Really good!
> Healthier feels good. And I feel stronger too.
> Not just muscle strength but you know I feel like
> I can do more and last longer doing things.

>> Whenever we encourage our kids to contribute in the kitchen, safety is always a priority. The best way to prevent an accident is to take a moment prior to starting any kitchen project and mentally go through where problem areas may exist. Kids can participate in this as well. Ask them, "Do you see anything that could be dangerous before we get started?" This will also give them confidence in their own safety.

Be Prepared

If a fire starts in your kitchen, you need to act fast and smart. Each type of fire gets treated differently, so you need to know what has caused the fire. Always keep a kitchen-specific fire extinguisher close by. (Type B is rated for grease and Type C is rated for electrical; combined ratings are also available.) And always keep baking soda within easy reach in the kitchen.

If your clothing catches on fire, stop, drop, and roll on the ground.

If you have a fire in the oven or microwave, close the door quickly. Turn off the oven. Don't open the door! The lack of oxygen should suffocate the flames.

If you have a fire in a cooking pan, quickly put a lid on it and move the pan off the burner. The lack of oxygen should stop the flames. If you can't put a lid on it, use your fire extinguisher. Aim at the base of the fire—not at the flames.

Never use water to put out grease fires! Water repels grease and can spread the fire by splattering the grease. Instead, throw lots of baking soda on it. (Never use flour.)

Do not swat at a fire with a towel, apron, or other clothing. You may fan the flames and spread the fire.

If the fire is spreading and you can't control it, get everyone out of the house and call 911! Keeping your stove and oven clean and free of debris and oils that might catch fire, as well as being aware of your surroundings, is the prevention necessary for a safe kitchen.

Kale Chips

This was a totally new thing for all of us to try, as we had never had kale before. It was good, and I can see making snack-bag portions of these to keep around for a healthy snack. I can also think of a couple of ideas to gussy these up even a little more, like adding curry or sesame seeds, but here is a basic recipe. This is another simple one that kids can easily handle on their own.

» 1 bag kale, rinsed and dried
» Olive oil
» Sea salt or kosher salt
» Parmesan or Asiago cheese

To prepare the kale, tear the leaves off the thick stems into bite-size pieces. Spread the kale out onto a cookie sheet. (You may need a couple of cookie sheets.)

Drizzle the smallest amount of olive oil on the leaves, then sprinkle with salt and cheese. This is where you can get a little creative!

Bake at 375°F for about 15 minutes, or until the kale is crispy and the edges are brown.

Let your meat rest after cooking? Why? I did all the work!

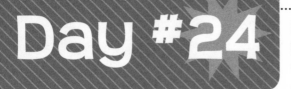

Day #24

Marshall: I get made fun of for being bigger than others. I think it's my weight that's holding me back, along with my genetics, but there are no excuses. I think it's my weight that's keeping me antisocial. So it's like a vicious cycle. I'm not social because I'm overweight, and I'm overweight because I'm not social and active.

Alex: When I was in the midst of my burnout stage of cooking at home, I asked the kids to each plan a meal twice a week with the idea that if they had control over what they were being served, they would eat it. We did this successfully for over a year. However, it stopped for two reasons. First of all, it was expensive. Oftentimes the things they picked were not on sale. And second of all, it did require some amount of organizing and discipline—God forbid you should miss their day; you would never hear the end of it.

Now I have learned through Marshall and Jordan that I can prepare a meal as I have in the past with all the negativity, or I can get them involved, which seems to be more positive than negative. And I don't mean just handing them the controls of the decisions but that they have to perform and follow through in that decision. This new concept of collaboration seems to be bringing peace to our household.

Tilapia

Day 24
Video 1

The low-fat flesh of the tilapia fish is white or sometimes pink. Tilapia is readily available, it's affordable, and it has a very mild taste. If you are looking to incorporate more fish into your diet, this fish is a good one to start with.

» Panko or homemade bread crumbs
» Lots of garlic powder
» Salt and pepper
» Parmesan cheese
» Tilapia fillets, defrosted
» Lemon juice
» Lemon wedges

Mix together the panko or bread crumbs, garlic powder, salt, pepper, and Parmesan cheese in a bowl.

Dip the fish fillets in lemon juice and dunk them into the bread crumb mixture. Spray a skillet with cooking spray and heat over very high heat. Cook the fish quickly on the hot skillet until the outside is crispy. Serve with the additional lemon wedges.

Watch Marshall prepare tilapia fillets.

Don't eat food just because it is cheap. It may be cheap for your body too, which winds up getting expensive later because of poor health. Eating cheap food means it's most likely heavily processed and has cheap, fake things in it. So if you eat that kind of stuff, you will be ingesting things that aren't good for you.

Check the shelf life of the packaged items you purchase. No matter how many preservatives they pack in, packaged foods can still expire, and they may not be the freshest unhealthy thing you want to taste. Even vacuum-sealed Meals Ready to Eat (MREs) can go bad.

Encouragement from a School Administrator

Marshall Reid's passion for educating others about good nutrition is contagious. As an administrator in the district where Marshall attends school, I have witnessed his efforts to implement a healthy food initiative at his elementary school. Marshall's organizational skills and commitment to healthy nutrition have already helped numerous children learn more about better eating habits. It is clear that Marshall's crusade is the leading edge of a growing national campaign to educate children and adults regarding the negative aspects of obesity. *Portion Size Me* is a timely and practical contribution to the growing literature on healthy eating for families in a fast-paced culture.

—Dr. Andy Bryan, Associate Superintendent,
    Curriculum & Instruction

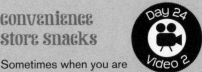

convenience store snacks

Day 24 Video 2

Sometimes when you are out and about and hungry, you just have to stop and grab a snack and a drink. Gas stations these days provide just about every piece of crud possible to entice you to pick something up. One day we stopped and investigated the snacks at a local gas station, trying to pick what we thought was the best. Nuts are usually a good choice, and our next favorite would be beef jerky. Both are a little pricier than a candy bar, but if you consider the nutritional value you get from them, they far outweigh something that is fake.

Marshall searches for the healthiest snacking options at his local gas station.

Preservatives are natural or man-made chemicals that are added to foods to keep them from spoiling. We actually "preserve" fresh foods ourselves every day by storing foods in the fridge or freezer. Slowly smoking fish or meats over burning coals is a method of preservation. Salting meats is an ancient technique that actually makes the meat resistant to bacteria. Many packaged foods we buy need a preserving agent to keep them from becoming rancid and to protect us against food-borne illnesses (e.g., food poisoning), which is why these preservatives are used. Natural preservatives that can be added to foods include salt and sugar and pickling. All additives, including preservatives, must be labeled on food packages. You may commonly see the word "preservative," followed by its additive number or name. For example, "preservative (220)" or "(sulphur dioxide)." This system, in theory, makes it easy to identify preservatives in foods. At the very least, you are reading the labels and beginning to recognize what is being used to increase the shelf life of your foods.

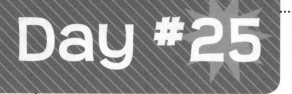

Day #25

Marshall: Not everyone is built for cooking. It's just like athletics: you're for it or not. People who are built for cooking can make bread and then mess up and be like, let's just try it again. People who aren't built for it mess up a little tiny bit but get very frustrated and say, "Ah, man, we have to start all over." I guess what I am trying to say is that it may not come easy to everyone. But if you are not so hard on yourself and be patient, it will come. 'Cause like my mom has been saying, "If you know better, do better." As in the choices of fuel to put in your body and the patience to cook.

Mom's note: Sounds like a life analogy here to me!

Sweet Potato Fries

If you like French fries, you will really like these sweet potato fries—even if you don't care for sweet potatoes. Give them a try. Consider one large sweet potato to be two servings. I like the skin on them, but you can use a vegetable peeler to remove it. Cut the potatoes into thin slices, or make them big and beefy like steak-house fries. Toss them in a small amount of olive oil, just so they are evenly coated, and sprinkle on Lawry's Seasoned Salt or regular salt and pepper. Place the fries in a baking dish—I like to use one of those clay Pampered Chef dishes—and bake at 400°F for about 25 minutes. (If your fries are thicker, you will have to cook them longer. Do not turn them while they're baking, or they may tear.) Then raise the temperature to 450°F and cook the fries for another 10 minutes, or until they're browned and crispy, just the way you like them.

Watch Marshall make sweet potato fries.

Alex: I fell off the wagon today. I was driving home from a tennis match (I had lost) and craved a cheeseburger. I indulged my craving, and afterward, I was so upset with myself for that decision. But then I told myself it was OK, and I tried to figure out why we do that to ourselves. Make a mistake and then beat ourselves up for it, that is. So I came up with an idea to help people with that type of situation.

Let's say that we have six opportunities to make food decisions in a day. Breakfast, lunch, dinner, and three snacks. Then let's add two opportunities for exercise, one for regular exercise and one for decisions like walking up stairs instead of using an elevator or parking farther away in a parking lot to increase walking. So that makes eight good decisions you can make in a day. Let's add two more decisions for the fluid decisions you make: drinking enough water, passing on sodas, etc. So in a day, you want to reach for a perfect ten good decisions. But if you hit a nine, is that a bad thing? No, not in my book! What if you are currently living at the two or three levels? You have a lot of room for improvement. What if you are at a constant eight? Can you look at those decision categories and see if you repeat the same two poor decisions? Make an adjustment there. If you look at it this way, it may prevent you from going through unreasonable swings of behavior.

I enjoy cooking, but I don't like having to wait for food to be done. You know you watch all those futuristic shows where they put one little piece of a seed in a microwave, and then you see a flash of light, you open the microwave, and there's a hamburger. I think that would be really cool, but at the same time, I think that would be really lame because you're not cooking, you're just sitting there. So if you are impatient like me, try reading a book or doing your homework while you wait for things to be done cooking.

My friend Terri said something funny the other day: "Ketchup is a condiment, not a base of a recipe!" She is a dental hygienist, and she followed that statement up with information about how much sugar is in ketchup, and how the sugar has been directly connected to contributing to cavities in children. I just pulled out a bottle from the fridge, and there it was on the label: high-fructose corn syrup and 4 grams of sugar per 1 tablespoon. Yikes. They really sneak it in there, don't they?

Food Pyramid: Steps to a Healthier You!

Be realistic: Make small changes over time in what you eat and the level of activity you do. After all, small steps often work better than giant leaps.

Be adventurous: Expand your tastes to enjoy a variety of foods and physical activities.

Be flexible: Go ahead and find your right balance between what you eat and the physical activity you do over several days. No need to worry about just one meal or one day.

Be sensible: Enjoy the foods you eat—just don't overdo it.

Be active: Walk the dog; don't just watch the dog walk.

—choosemyplate.gov

Stuffed Bell Peppers

Day 25
Videos 2-4

» 1 pound lean ground beef or lean turkey
» 1 yellow onion, diced
» Lot of garlic, crushed
» Salt and pepper
» A few sweet mini bell peppers, chopped (optional)
» 6 servings brown rice
» 4 whole bell peppers
» 1 to 2 cans stewed or diced tomatoes (check ingredients)
» Parmesan cheese

In a large skillet, brown the ground meat with the onion, garlic, salt and pepper, and mini bell peppers until the beef is cooked through.

Cook the rice, following the package directions, and set aside.

Clean and hollow out the bell peppers and blanch them (see page 71) in boiling water for about 1 minute.

Mix the rice and tomatoes into the beef mixture and taste. If the mixture is too dry, add the second can of tomatoes. But you don't want it too wet either, just nice and moist.

Place the bell peppers in a baking tray with high sides. Stuff each bell pepper with the beef and rice mixture, and then spread what remains of the mixture around the peppers to help them stay standing up. Sprinkle with Parmesan, and bake at 350°F degrees for about 20 minutes.

See Marshall prepare his stuffed bell peppers in these videos.

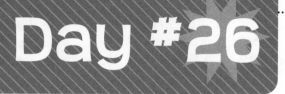

Day #26

Taco salad

How is this different from a regular old taco salad? First, you get your children involved with making it. Second, it's about using reduced-fat sour cream and cheeses. And lastly, it's about adding new and flavorful items that you may normally skip over, such as:

- » Cilantro, chopped
- » Chayote, diced (this is a member of the squash and cucumber family)
- » Black beans
- » Pickled eggs
- » Red radish, diced
- » Lime juice
- » Corn
- » Colorful peppers, diced

Consider not adding any meat to it, or using cooked ground chicken, or a medley of beans. Add different lettuces and maybe a few leaves of spinach.

Layer everything in a large bowl or have family members assemble their own in individual bowls.

The overall point is to introduce new things and flavors. You can do it all at once or slowly add new items each time you prepare this dish while at the same time removing unwanted or unhealthy things, like the fried taco shell bowl or chips.

Watch Marshall assemble his favorite taco salad.

Marshall: I don't understand why restaurants serve so much bad stuff. We have this book *Eat This, Not That*, and when you look at all the fat and calories in some of the food at restaurants, it's just amazing. What happened to good food in those places? I think people would eat out more and support restaurants if their food was better for you. But I bet a lot of people don't know how bad it is for you. It doesn't have to be that way. We have remade some of these recipes here at home in a healthier way, and they taste just as good.

Alex: As a child growing up and cooking for my mom, I always viewed the process as a chore. As a young adult in school and having only myself to take care of, I viewed cooking as a necessary evil. But when my family came together, I viewed cooking as the measure of my love. It was my way of showing them how much I love them by thinking creatively and considering what would make them happy.

As I said before, I broke that cycle when I let the culmination of a busy schedule and my family's lack of appreciation steer me away from my loving efforts. But I wonder how many other parents out there provide food to please or as a measure of love. I don't mean that they are using food as bribery or a reward, a topic I have also addressed. But rather, I wonder how many parents actually feel a sense of fulfillment and completion when the meal is provided. And if that is the case, are we choosing the healthiest of balanced foods to also make our children stronger, or are we offering meals to fill our kids' souls in an unhealthy, unbalanced way?

I want to be a dad someday. And I want to be able to do things with my kids. PSM is helping me learn that I can do more activities and be able to teach them things.

> A whisk, a spatula, a wooden spoon, a colander, and a paring knife. These would be the kitchen essentials to gift to your child today to encourage him or her to help you in the kitchen.

Tips for Portion Control from the Centers for Disease Control and Prevention (CDC)

Portion control when eating in. To minimize the temptation of second and third helpings when eating at home, serve food on individual plates instead of putting the serving dishes on the table. Keeping the excess food out of reach may discourage overeating.

Portion control in front of the TV. When eating or snacking in front of the TV, put the amount that you plan to eat into a bowl or container instead of eating straight from the package. It's easy to overeat when your attention is focused on something else.

Go ahead, spoil your dinner. We learned as children not to snack before a meal for fear of "spoiling our dinner." Well, it's time to forget that old rule. If you feel hungry between meals, eat a healthy snack, like a piece of fruit or small salad, to avoid overeating during your next meal.

Be aware of large packages. For some reason, the larger the package, the more people consume from it without realizing it. To minimize this effect:

Divide up the contents of one large package into several smaller containers to help avoid over-consumption.

Don't eat straight from the package. Instead, serve the food in a small bowl or container.

Out of sight, out of mind. People tend to consume more when they have easy access to food. Make your home a "portion friendly zone."

Replace the candy dish with a fruit bowl.

Store especially tempting foods, like cookies, chips, or ice cream, out of immediate eyesight, like on a high shelf or in the back of the freezer. Move the healthier food to the front at eye level.

When buying in bulk, store the excess in a place that's not convenient to get to, such as a high cabinet or in the back of the pantry.

Garbage in a skillet

Day 26 — Video 2

We have been serving this breakfast for years. Basically, it is the leftovers from the week thrown into a cast-iron skillet with a diced potato and a couple of eggs. Have some leftover stuffed bell pepper filling from Day 25? Sure, toss it in. Leftover lunch meat or London broil from Day 23? Why not? Extra onion and bell peppers? Of course! Just chop them all up and get them cooking. When the potatoes are cooked and everything else is heated, toss in a couple of eggs and scramble it all together. Top with a bit of shredded low-fat cheese, and voilà! So much better for you than doughnuts!

In Mexico, the word "taco" is a generic term, like the English word "sandwich." Like a sandwich, a taco can be made with just about anything.

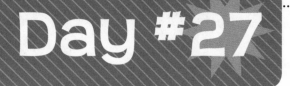
Day #27

Marshall: I like how this is working out. We are having more and more subscribers on YouTube, and I think they are listening to what we are saying. I am getting out to people. I have had a lot of really positive comments. It makes me feel like we are helping people. Some commenters have said that they have kids with weight issues and that they are inspired by us. That's cool. I like that!

Alex: I believe we have discovered an unknown talent of Marshall's. All of the videos are done with my iPhone camera and are not rehearsed. We've only needed to do a few retakes due to distractions from friends or his big sister. Marshall is quite at ease in front of the camera, and I am impressed with how clear and appropriately animated he is. Perhaps he has a future as a TV weatherman in front of him.

More seriously, this experience has opened my eyes to the need to really investigate things outside of our normal comforts and patterns. To reach out and explore new life and civilizations. To boldly go...I digress. This experience was quite accidental, but it reveals the requirement there is for a parent to be open-minded, try new things, and discover what makes a kid feel enthused as a leader.

Nutty Dessert

Marshall was looking for a sweet treat. He took a handful of cashews and put them in a bowl, drizzled a little honey over the top, and then heated his snack in the microwave for about 30 seconds. Delicious!

> Switching to brown rice is really easy for me, and now I am pretty comfortable with whole-wheat noodles. Whole-wheat bread? I need to work on that longer. You just gotta do it slowly or you will set in your head that you don't like it, forever.

Marshall talks about making the switch to whole-wheat bread.

Switching to whole-wheat products can be difficult at first, with wheat's hearty, nutty bite. But don't let it hinder you from starting. One idea is to switch gradually by mixing half of your noodles, half of your rice servings, and half of your bread with the whole-grain versions.

Awe Nuts!

Nuts are various dry fruits that generally consist of an edible kernel enclosed in a shell that can range from medium-hard, thin, and brittle to woody and tough. Botanically speaking, some foods we know as nuts are actually seeds (such as the Brazil nut) or legumes (like the peanut). Among the more popular of the other nuts are almonds, cashews, chestnuts, macadamias, pecans, pistachios, pine nuts, and walnuts. Most nuts are sold both shelled and unshelled. Shelled nuts come in many forms, including blanched or not, whole, halved, chopped, sliced, or minced. Nuts are high in calcium, folic acid, magnesium, potassium, vitamin E, and fiber.

The germ, bran, and endosperm

make up the three parts of a whole grain. Every grain starts out as a whole grain and gets broken down into parts during milling. Even after milling, if all three parts are kept in their original proportions, they can still be considered whole grains.

Shortcut Pesto

Day 27
Videos 1-3

The kids like a dish similar to Day 14's whole-wheat noodles with ham and tomatoes. This time it's whole-wheat noodles with fresh garden basil and olive oil, and it's almost like a pesto. To prepare it, they mince basil and add it to a couple tablespoons of olive oil and lots of minced garlic in a sauté pan. It takes them just about as long to make the shortcut pesto sauce as it takes to cook the noodles.

Traditionally, pesto is made with pine nuts and cheese in the mixture, but we found that our simpler recipe is just as good. If you are growing your own basil and you have a lot of pesto made, you can freeze it in an ice cube tray. Once the cubes are frozen, remove them from the tray and place them in freezer bags in the serving portions you desire. When you are ready to use the pesto, thaw the cubes at a room temperature for a bit, mix the sauce well, and add it to your recipe. You can also use pesto as a sandwich spread, on crackers for a snack, and even as a veggie dip.

Watch Marshall make shortcut pesto.

What sound does a peanut make when it sneezes? Cashew!

Day #28

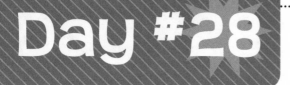

Marshall: You guys! You need to step out of your comfort zones and try new things. If you don't ever try anything new, you're gonna be stuck in your limit zone that you're already in for the rest of your life. Are you going to be a control freak? You know, if a baby never tried milk, then he may never drink it. So you gotta try new things now, not when you're 103. You have to do it when you're young so that you develop taste buds for it.

When I have been at farmers' markets and in Chinatown (NYC), looking at all those exotic fruits, it's quite amazing because they have so many different things, things I've never heard of. So we have bought a few and tried them and they are pretty good.

Go ahead, step out of your comfort zone. Ya know, my sister likes to eat those tamarinds. They taste like bitter melon to me, but at least I tried it. And she tried them and likes them. See what I mean?

Unique Fruits

» Cherimoya
» Tomatillo
» Young coconut
» Meyer lemon
» Kumquat
» Pummelo
» Star fruit
» Ugli fruit
» Litchi (often found canned)

Have you heard of any of these fruits? I bet you could find one or two at your local grocery store and even more available at a specialty store. Pick one up and introduce it to your family. You may be surprised that fruits that are commonly eaten in other countries but not necessarily in the United States are quite tasty. Their prices and availability fluctuate just like common fruits. I'm only suggesting you look to widen your variety not empty your pocket book.

There are so many unique and delish fruits available at local markets and grocery stores. Go out and try a new fruit today!

Watch Marshall try out some new fruits as he explores Chinatown in New York City.

Alex: Here we are at Day 28 and Marshall has lost 11 pounds and about 2 body-mass index points. I have lost 6 pounds. Is this really a valid idea? Cutting back on portion sizes; pausing to contemplate what fuel we want in our bodies; and returning to the kitchen to make meals, have conversations, and spend time together as a family? I know that the change in harmony and peace in our household is unmistakable. But we really have only done simple things. Those five Portion Size Me goals don't seem that drastic and yet here we are smiling for so many reasons. I believe we can sustain this and make it our new lifelong habit.

The weight loss isn't the measure for me now. It's all the growing we are doing together. It's the talking and planning and commitment and smiles. It's the questions and discoveries and answers. It's the sunshine heating beads of sweat on our skin as we catch our breath from one activity and plan our next physical adventure. It's standing in the produce section of the market and looking at all the colors and textures and discussing our next steps. That feels like success and I am so proud of us!

PSM has brought out the best in us! So many are proud of us. Strangers are sending us some emails from our videos. My aunt is telling me I am looking good. We have accomplished a lot, but we want to go farther. We are not letting our shapes shape our lives!

Go on a hunt at the grocery store with your child and see who can find any of the listed fruits first! Whoever identifies a fruit first gets to research how to eat it and serve it to the rest of the family.

There are about two thousand fruits across the globe, but only about 10 percent are used in the Western world, in part because many fruits are poisonous to humans. How did humans first learn what was poisonous or safe? It is commonly believed that early humans mostly observed how animals behaved around foods, watching whether or not they avoided them.

Lekvar

Plums, apricots, prunes, and figs are fruits that don't seem to be eaten very much in the States but are used quite a bit in many European countries. One way to utilize these fruits is to make lekvar with them. You can make this thick jam from a single variety of fruit or a combination thereof. All you do is put the dried fruits in a pot with a little water and a hearty squeeze of lemon juice, and cook it down for about 30 minutes, mashing the fruit when you stir it. You don't want all the water to evaporate, so you may need to add a bit more to keep the fruit from sticking to the bottom of the pot. Then add some brown sugar to sweeten it enough to your liking. Cook for another 10 minutes and then puree in a blender.

We like to spread this on a piece of sourdough bread or some sliced apples, much the way you might put peanut butter on apples. The lekvar will keep in your fridge for several weeks.

Body mass index (BMI) is a number calculated from a person's weight and height. BMI provides a reliable but basic indicator of body fat for most people, and it is used to screen for weight categories that may lead to health problems. The CDC has a BMI measurement calculator available online for adults and for youth.

Watch Marshall talk about how important it is to read ingredients.

Day 28
Video 2

Track

Helpful Hint!

Meat needs to rest for several minutes after cooking. This is because it continues to cook on the inside even after you have removed it from its heat source. If you cut into the meat too early, all the juices will run out and you'll be left with a tougher piece of meat. After the meat begins to cool, it holds in its juices and you'll get more flavors.

Your Journey!

Fun Fact!

Plunging foods into rapidly boiling water for a brief time is called blanching. The reason to do this is to only partially cook the food, improve its flavor and color, or to make the skin easier to peel off. After you remove the food from the hot water, immediately rinse it in cold water or submerge it in a bowl of ice water. This stops any additional cooking that may happen, and it's called shocking the food.

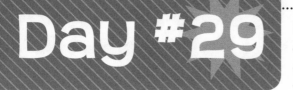

Day #29

Marshall: *I have noticed that when I am actually in the kitchen making an omelet or something, cracking an egg, hands touching the food, smelling it all, and feeling all the different textures, when I finish, I find I don't actually eat as much—which is good. Prepping my food helps control my hunger. I'm not starving or anything. I think it's because you get those sensations and satisfactions you want from the food in the cooking process.*

Alex: Yesterday I commented in a very upbeat way about our success. But I think we still need to work harder to change our behaviors to make them more permanent and ingrained into our souls. I can see that, even now, it would still be quite easy to slip back to the "easy" habits.

Tortilla Soup

This is an easy dish to make, and it is great to pack as a lunch for school or work. It's very satisfying and flavorful.

- » 1 whole chicken, cooked in a large stock pot of water and deboned (keep the resulting chicken stock)
- » Lots of celery, chopped
- » 1 onion, diced
- » 1 bell pepper, chopped
- » 1 can of Rotel tomatoes and peppers
- » 1 large can of diced tomatoes, drained
- » Can of beans, any variety
- » 1 can enchilada sauce
- » 1 can hominy
- » Any other leftover peppers, chopped (We had 3 red mini bell peppers.)
- » Lots of fresh garlic or garlic powder
- » Salt and pepper
- » Few dashes of cumin
- » 6 servings of brown rice, uncooked
- » Bunch of cilantro, washed and minced
- » Fresh lime, washed and sliced
- » Avocados, diced
- » 2 handfuls corn tortilla chips, crushed into a bowl

Place the chicken into a pot with the stock it was cooked in, and add everything up to and including the brown rice. Let the mixture simmer for 10 minutes while you prepare the remaining items to be served as garnishes.

Taste the soup and season accordingly, and then serve with the cilantro, lime, avocado, and chips as garnishes. Delightfully filling and simple.

We are filled with hope and feeling good. We want to tap into that, harness it, and drive forward! Just being aware of how we feel and focusing on the positives will help us remember those feelings and want to have them again. That is our strategy.

The choice to be healthy is up to you. If you are feeling good, then you should continue with what makes you feel good so that you stay feeling good. If you are feeling not so good, then you can change that. It's all about you! **Jordan explains this in a video here.**

Day 29
Video 1

Aunt Pilar's Enchiladas

Aunt Pilar, my older sister, loves to cook! She loves to concoct and create rich and layered flavors. We have nicknamed her Aunt Pepper because she also loves to season things with pepper—a lot of pepper! We all benefit from her cooking explorations because she gets so excited about her idea and putting it together that she overindulges in quantity and cooks for an army. That is a benefit to us because we are often surprised with a meal in the refrigerator we did not expect. Here she shares with you her healthier enchiladas.

» 3 boneless chicken breasts
» Salt and pepper
» Lots of garlic powder
» 2 pinches of cumin, divided
» 1 teaspoon chicken bouillon or the equivalent of bouillon cubes
» 3 cups brown rice
» 1 (10-ounce) can fat-free cream of chicken soup
» 1 (8-ounce) container low-fat Greek or plain yogurt, divided
» 2 (10-ounce) cans diced tomatoes, drained

» 1 can diced chiles
» 1 (14-ounce) bag 2 percent milk shredded mozzarella cheese
» Whole-wheat tortillas
» 1 (23-ounce) jar chunky marinara sauce
» Cheddar cheese
» 1 (15-ounce) can reduced-sodium black beans, drained and rinsed
» 2 scallions, diced
» 2 medium tomatoes, diced
» 2 tablespoons light, zesty Italian dressing

Season the chicken breasts on both sides with the salt and pepper, garlic powder, and 1 pinch of cumin. Spray a baking pan with cooking spray, and then place the chicken in the pan. Bake at 400°F for 20 minutes. Remove the chicken from the oven, cut it into strips, and place it back in the oven to cook another 10 minutes. Take the chicken out, cool a little bit, and shred it with a fork. Set aside.

In a saucepan, add the chicken bouillon to water and prepare the rice according to the package directions. Set aside.

In a pot, combine the chicken soup, yogurt, canned diced tomatoes, chiles, and mozzarella cheese. Stir and heat thoroughly. Then add the shredded chicken and rice. Thoroughly mix together over low heat.

Place the filling mixture down center of a tortilla, fold the ends over, and place each enchilada seam side down in a pan. Repeat, filling the pan with tortillas side by side until the pan is full.

In a saucepan, heat together the marinara sauce and a pinch of cumin, and spoon over the enchiladas. Sprinkle lightly with Cheddar cheese. Place in a 350°F oven and bake for 15 minutes.

Meanwhile, mix the black beans, scallions, and tomatoes together and toss with the Italian dressing. Sprinkle the black bean salsa on top of the finished enchiladas. Serve with a dollop of low-fat Greek yogurt over the top.

Day #30

Paella

- » 2 pounds skinless chicken pieces (This can be boneless, skinless chicken breasts that you cut into small chunks, or you can boil two whole chickens and debone them for the meat. The latter is less expensive but more time consuming.)
- » Splash of olive oil
- » Dash of salt and pepper
- » 2 cups chicken broth
- » 1 cup whole-grain rice, uncooked
- » 1 onion, cut into wedges
- » 2 or 3 celery stalks, chopped
- » 1 small jar pimientos
- » Lots of garlic, minced
- » ½ teaspoon oregano
- » ⅛ teaspoon saffron (This spice is fairly expensive and does add a unique flavor, however the dish is great without it as well.)
- » 1 can nonmarinated artichoke hearts, diced
- » 1 small bag frozen, cooked shelled shrimp

In a very large skillet with a cover, cook the chicken in oil with salt and pepper over medium heat until brown, about 10 minutes.

Add the broth, rice, onion, celery, pimiento, garlic, oregano, and saffron. Bring to a boil, then reduce the heat and simmer, covered, for 15 minutes.

Add the artichoke hearts and shrimp and cook for another 5 minutes. Serve.

Marshall: A lot of different foreign cultures don't have as many restaurants as the United States has, and their families eat together more too. Look at the samurai. They are probably the most honorable of people I have read about. I use this idea because the Japanese government was trying to get rid of the samurai, who would not use guns; the samurai thought you were being a coward by fighting your enemy from far away. Good food is like the samurai. It honors the body. The gun is like fast food. It dishonors the body. It is all about honor for your mind and body—that is what the samurai felt.

Alex: Eating together is a social event, but we often seem too exhausted to be social with our loved ones at the end of the day. Our meals become less wholesome when we eat separately in front of a TV screen, computer monitor, or even a cell phone. We seem to need a quick fix of some type of cheap entertainment rather than thoughtful and active engagement with our loved ones. Taking the time to share in the ritual of eating and talking with each person about what is going on in his or her life is a lot more than a way to "catch up on the news." It is also a time to share opinions, teach your children how to communicate, teach them how to listen, and show them that they can be heard and have their own voices.

I want to be what I picture myself to be! Like a cop or a football player. They both have to be strong and agile. I want to be what other people picture me to be! I feel that a lot of the expectations are high for my age and different than they should be. It will be hard to make both things happen but if you put your mind to anything you can make it happen.

PORTION SIZE ME

> Disconnect from your unwanted habits in life and start anew! Tap into your new wanted habits and live your life to its fullest.

Discrimination

You nailed a phone interview for a new job. But once you meet your prospective boss in person, things go downhill quickly. Either your meeting is cut short or you're abruptly told the position has been filled.

The scenario is an all-too-familiar one for a number of overweight people who have experienced weight-based discrimination in the workforce. While many victims of the bias have suspected their appearance has been hurting their careers, there are new studies out looking at decades' worth of research that show just how pervasive the problem is.

Saffron, made from the three lone little stigmas (threads) of a crocus flower, is the world's most expensive spice. The flowers must be hand picked, and it takes over fourteen thousand of them to make one ounce of spice. Saffron has been used for thousands of years in cooking, dying fabrics, and medicine. It is written that saffron was the most frequently forged commodity. Fortunately, a little goes a long way with this potent little beauty.

Flan

This is an incredibly popular dessert in Spain and other countries around the world. We have not provided many desserts in this book because when we do, we want them to be *good* and that is *bad*. That's the point. You can enjoy anything and everything you want every once in a while. Flan every night would *not* be an example of moderation.

- » 1 cup sugar
- » 4 eggs (Ours are from our hens.)
- » 1 (14-ounce) can sweetened condensed milk
- » 1 (12-ounce) can evaporated milk
- » 1½ tablespoons vanilla extract
- » Pinch of salt

In a medium saucepan, melt the sugar over medium heat until it is liquefied and golden in color. Keep an eye on this, or the sugar will burn quickly. Carefully pour the hot syrup into a 9-inch round glass baking dish, turning the dish to evenly coat the bottom and sides. *Danger: do not get hot syrup on your skin or try to taste it with your finger. Hot sugar will burn you.* Set the dish aside.

In a large bowl, beat the eggs with an electric mixer. Beat in the condensed milk, evaporated milk, vanilla extract, and salt until smooth. Pour the egg mixture into the baking dish. Cover with aluminum foil.

Bake in a 350°F oven for 60 minutes. Let the flan cool completely. Carefully run a butter knife around the edges of the dish, place a large plate on top of it, and invert it so that the flan comes out of the dish.

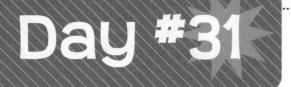

Day #31

Marshall: We celebrated! We went over to Aunt Pilar's house and set off a ton of fireworks. Uncle Robert cooked fish he had caught all summer long and made hush puppies and cornbread. It was a delightful evening and fun for all.

I feel like I accomplished something great! I feel excited to continue more. I want to be able to run and I want to get rid of my belly. You have come this far. Don't quite now! If you're tempted to quit, don't. Because this is for you. Keep going. Don't give up. It's like running a marathon: if you quit, you can never say you ran a marathon!

Alex: These thirty-one days have truly been amazing. How we each feel about ourselves and how we feel about each other is foreign. But foreign is an outside source and this is driven from inside the walls of our house. So what is it if it is not foreign? New? Well, that is a boring word. The proper word escapes me but I do know that we must continue to positively change our behaviors. Anyway today we celebrate the completion of our commitment and the continuation of a commitment to ourselves.

Edamame Succotash

We brought this fresh side dish to the party to complement the fish and hush puppies.

- » 4 splashes olive oil
- » 1 red onion, diced
- » Couple garlic cloves, minced
- » 1 (8-ounce) package frozen and shelled edamame
- » 2 cups fresh-cut corn kernels (about 3 ears) or frozen corn, thawed
- » 2 large ripe tomatoes, diced
- » Dash salt
- » Dash freshly ground pepper
- » Some chopped fresh basil or cilantro

Add olive oil to skillet and warm up. Add onion and garlic and brown quickly for about 1 minute. Add edamame and corn. Cook for another minute. Add tomatoes, salt, pepper, and your herb of choice and cook quickly for another minute. Remove from stove and cool before serving.

Are you feeling all right now? Do you want to keep that going or do you want to put that down and be a couch potato? By the way, I suggest the first one.

If you have siblings in the kitchen trying to help you, and they are anything like mine, being the ring leader to manage those alternating steps in recipes can cause your blood to boil. Kick one out of the kitchen and then start over by alternating one kid for one meal. You're not playing favorites, just keeping your blood pressure down.

Celebration: A time or program of special events and entertainment in honor of something.

Watch the kids thirty-one-day celebratory finale at Aunt Pilar's house.

Day 31
Video 1

End of the First Month

Let's put aside the food, health, and nutrition conversation for a moment. Our family has just done something totally outside of our "normal" box. And we have done it for a month. That's like forever for our household! We have been happy, excited, positive, and incredibly real with each other. We have shared, explored, and connected. I believe Marshall and I have tapped into our deepest character building blocks. And I can confirm, at least from my perspective, that we have a new sense of what the future has to offer us. I am sure the improved nutrition and sense of health play a role, but I also believe that this project has put us on a path that helps us feel secure and confident with ourselves and with each other. That security leads us to liking each other better and enjoying each other as we continue down the path. Dan is following us from half a world away. I cannot even imagine how he feels…perhaps isolated and alone. But my soul tells me that he does not look at the videos from the kids with sorrow and jealousy for not being involved but with pride and eagerness to come home and be a part of our renewed sense of energy. Jordan seems less teenagerish to me and more like a lovely young lady. Perhaps that is the result of better nutrition or the good feelings we are having with each other, or both. Regardless, I cannot deny the shift in the Reid household.

To this point our videos and recipes have been a little sporadic and may not be practical for everyone as we were enjoying a summer break and were not suffering from strict time pressures. So we thought about adding another thirty days to be a little more specific and focus on one meal at a time. Ten days of breakfasts, ten days of school lunches, and ten days of affordable dinners. Then by having those and our previous efforts under our belts and on a list, we will all be empowered with more choices when we are facing the ticking of the clock.

Ten Days of Breakfasts

Why have we decided to do ten days of breakfasts? Because typically it's the hardest meal for our family to create and enjoy. We have such varied morning habits. Jordan does not eat in the mornings. She needs several hours of awake time before her tummy gets rolling. It doesn't matter what you give her; she won't eat it. Dan and I are hungry about an hour after we wake, or after a morning workout. Marshall rolls out of bed hungry. But not only is it our schedules, and our natural internal feeding clocks, it's what we eat as well. None of us have been interested much in cereals, hot or cold. And who has the time to make eggs Benedict on busy school mornings? We thought we would do the ten days of breakfasts to force ourselves to look into our food culture and our choices, and open up more possibilities for us.

Ten Days of Breakfasts

Breakfast Day #1

Marshall: I guess I never thought about breakfast except as, you know, the traditional breakfast foods, like eggs and sausage, biscuits and gravy. My mom asked me the other day about having leftovers for breakfast. I thought that was weird. Then she told me I was food prejudiced because I only wanted breakfast stuff. I don't know why. That's just what I have always thought. I mean, we have had fruit too. But I wouldn't want an enchilada for breakfast. I mean it's just not right.

Blowing Out Eggs

Day 1
Video 1

This is a craft project instead of a recipe because we wanted to share some ideas to be joyful with and around food. What I mean is that you don't always have to eat it. There can be joy in deciding on food, purchasing food, creating dishes, and *playing* with food objects. Like painting a pinecone with peanut butter and hanging it outside for the birds and squirrels. You can have fun and joy with food. So, have you ever blown out an egg? If you ever did as a child, then now is the time to bring back that old-fashioned favorite. It's a great way to get kids busy doing something in the kitchen.

First, thoroughly wash a raw egg and use a safety pin or needle to poke a hole in one end of the shell. Poke another hole in the other end about twice as large, something a little larger than the tip of a ballpoint pen. Now, lean over a bowl, blow really hard through the small-hole end, and blow the contents out of the large-hole end. It'll take a bit of work but it's good for your lungs! Then rinse the egg and dry it. From here you can use acrylic paints and paint the eggs, use them to decorate around the bottom of plants, or even write messages on them like "You're Eggstra Special," and give them as gifts.

Watch Marshall make blow-out eggs in the Reid kitchen.

Alex: Here we are now concentrating on breakfasts and a shift has occurred in my thoughts and planning. For the first time ever, it occurs to me that one's body has been void of food energy now for roughly ten hours. It (your body) is ready to perform for you for the entire busy day. Why would you ever load it up first thing with sugary, nutritionally void fuel? A doughnut? Starchy, heavy cinnamon rolls? It would be like emptying the tank on your car and then filling it with bad gasoline that may have debris and water in it. It will run all day, maybe, but it will be coughing and shaking and sputtering along.

My friend Adam and I discovered a really lazy way to make scrambled eggs, and even if you don't want to be lazy, it's fun to do this. Add eggs in a small bowl and whip with a whisk until well blended. Spray a dinner plate with light cooking oil (not entirely necessary). Add eggs onto the plate, careful that it doesn't spill over sides. Cook in the microwave for three minutes or until done. You end up with a thin egg omelet like a tortilla that you can eat plain or use as a wrap for other things.

PORTION SIZE ME

Use your leftover blown-out eggs to create decorations for Easter, the 4th of July, Halloween, Thanksgiving, or for any event. After you have blown out the eggs, wash them and let them dry completely. Then pull out the craft box. Lightly sketch your design on the egg and paint with acrylic paints. You can decorate them as gifts or for any holiday. Think of a basket of eggs all painted with red, white, and blue flags. How about a basket of eggs painted like jack-o-lanterns? Who says eggs are just for Easter?

Green Eggs and Ham

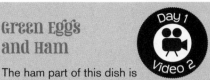

The ham part of this dish is lunch meat gently warmed in a skillet. In another skillet, scramble some eggs with diced broccoli, spinach, asparagus, or even shredded Brussels sprouts with a little low-fat Cheddar cheese and salt and pepper. Roll the cooked egg mixture into the ham slice like a burrito. Another option to make the eggs green is to make a smoothie out of the vegetables using a blender and tell the kids to think of it as healthy food coloring.

See Marshall talk about his green eggs.

Salmonella is bacteria that can cause diarrheal illness in humans. They are microscopic living creatures that pass from the feces of people or animals to other people or other animals.

The *Salmonella* family includes over 2,300 serotypes of bacteria, which are one-celled organisms too small to be seen without a microscope. Some of these bacteria cause no symptoms in animals but can make people sick, and vice versa. If present in food, the bacteria does not usually affect the taste, smell, or appearance of the food. It's very important to thoroughly wash your hands when working with food to help prevent illness.

You may notice a difference between mass-produced, store-bought eggs; fresh farm eggs; and everything in between to include cage-free, all natural feed, and free-range labels on eggs. You may find thick and thin shells, bright and firm yolks, or opaque and "relaxed" yolks. These variations are a direct result of the hen's diet and environment.

How did the egg get up the mountain? It scrambled up!

Breakfast Day #2

Marshall: I have noticed and heard some kids say they don't have breakfast before school. Sometimes I see them eating a breakfast bar or cookie. Sometimes I see them eat at school, but I know they don't serve the best stuff there. I much prefer to have breakfast at home. That is where you are supposed to have your first meal, and I like how it starts my day. My sister doesn't eat much breakfast. I bet she is cranky in the classroom. Thank goodness I am younger than her and don't have to be in the same class.

Alex: Marshall has mentioned high-fructose corn syrup several times in some of his videos. I wanted to clarify, on his behalf, that we are not against HFCS or other sugars. We have learned a little bit about the economics of sugar, and the fact of the matter is, we all like sugar. What we are advocating, however, is that everyone understands how much they are taking in and that each person actually chooses to consume sugar or HFCS instead of it being hidden in our food. That is the "pause" in PSM. Taking the time to read the ingredients and make a conscious and active decision in your choices. Cooking from scratch in the kitchen is the foundation of your nutritional fuel. Reading the ingredients of packaged items empowers you to not sabotage all the efforts you have made in the kitchen.

Broiled Grapefruit

Day 2
Video 1

Grapefruit seems to be viewed as an old-fashioned food, and quite honestly, I think Jordan was the only one in our family who liked it. But once we tried grapefruit this way, it opened the door to the rest of the family liking the tart fruit as well. In lieu of loading tons of sugar on it to take away the unbearable tartness, we tried putting half a grapefruit under the broiler and using just a small amount of sugar. Warming it up seems to bring out more of the natural sweetness, and the broiler gives it warmth that seems more comforting in the morning. Also, preparing a grapefruit can be a fun and quick activity for a young'un to do in the morning. You can use a regular paring knife and a teaspoon, but a grapefruit knife really helps out.

Marshall demonstrates how to use a grapefruit knife.

Have you ever seen a bent knife? Well, they make one for grapefruits. The tip of it is curled under. I think it's pretty cool that someone invented a bent knife.

I am not a proponent of getting kids to eat things at all costs by describing something as a breakfast cookie or turning a fruit-on-the-bottom yogurt upside down onto a plate and calling it a breakfast sundae. I think that does a disservice to their future decision-making abilities. A better option is to get them to help you in the kitchen. That automatically invests them to liking or at least trying what they've helped prepare.

The first recorded accounts of sugar come from the Pacific islands of Polynesia. It is thought to have spread from there to India and then farther to the Middle East over several centuries. Arab invaders of Persia (modern-day Iran) found the sweet substance and carried it back west with them. During the Middle Ages, Western Crusaders returning to Europe spoke of the sweetener that they experienced on their travels in the Arab lands.

Christopher Columbus is credited with introducing sugar to the Americas when he brought sugar cane plants to the Dominican Republic. The plants flourished in the climate and soon were spread throughout the Caribbean Islands. From there, they moved to South America in the 1600s and then to the United States around 1700.

Because sugar is a labor-intensive crop to grow, refine, and transport, it was always in short supply and was highly sought after. This, along with governmental taxation, made sugar very expensive. The people who could afford it stored it in a lockable "sugar chest" to protect their investment.

The expense of importing sugar led some to look for other sources of sweeteners. By the early 1800s, the sugar beet had been identified as a source, and by the 1880s it had overtaken sugar cane as the main source of sugar in the Western world.

In the mid-1950s, a new sweetener emerged on the market. Through scientific research, it was found that corn syrup could be modified and its glucose converted to fructose. This made the corn syrup, which at the time was a low-grade sweetener, as sweet, or even sweeter, than real sugar. Because the United States has a huge surplus of corn, it also made it cheap to produce. From the 1970s to the late 1990s, high-fructose corn syrup replaced real sugar as the primary sweetener in the U.S. market.

Hot Cereal

As a family, we've never really enjoyed cold cereal—thankfully, that is one thing we did do right. But with Coco Wheat, Cream of Wheat, oatmeal, porridge, gruel, Malt-O-Meal, and Cream of Rice available, whatever happened to hot cereal in the morning? And I don't mean the kinds with the colorful packaging and inserts of rubbery cartoon characters. So many nutritious and yummy items can be put into hot cereals to round them out and make them very interesting. You could even toss in some of the trail mix we make in Lunch Day 5. I am just trying to remind you of some wholesome and long-lost breakfast favorites. Another option: if you have a favorite healthy cold cereal, try it with warm milk instead of cold milk.

As well as being used as a sweetener, sugar is also used as a preservative, retarding microbial growth. For example, sugar helps to hinder the growth of bacteria in jam and syrups. It can also be used as an additive to achieve a certain kind of texture. Sometimes it's added to accelerate fermentation or to change the boiling or freezing point of a dish.

Breakfast Day #3

Right now, breakfasts have leaner meat and healthy fruit. I used to eat hash, canned roast beef hash. We looked at the fat and there were over 100 grams of fat. And I was eating the whole can. And you know, it was just nasty. I have really changed on the types of foods I eat at breakfast, and I am really proud of myself for that change.

Alex: I wonder how many households today have a juice reamer in their kitchen. It seems like such a grandmotherly tool. Why not have one, though? I find them in abundance in my antiquing journeys, but when I was younger, I remember always wanting an electric juicer. A juice reamer is such a simple and handy tool to have, and it provides direct and immediate satisfaction from making fresh juice (children in particular love it).

Chocolate Chip Popovers

Day 3
Video 1

» 2 eggs
» 1 cup milk
» 1 cup flour
» Two pinches of salt
» Dark chocolate chips

Crack the eggs into a bowl. Add the milk and beat with an electric mixer until blended.

Add the flour and salt, and stir with a spoon. Don't worry if a few lumps in the batter remain.

Pour a bit of the batter into greased muffin tins. Place about 4 dark chocolate chips on top of each muffin, and then place a bit more batter on top of the chocolate chips. Do not fill the muffin tins more than half full.

Place the tins in a cold oven. Turn the oven to 450°F and bake for 30 minutes. *Do not open the door and peek, as the popovers may pop and deflate.*

Serve hot, as soon as the popovers have cooled slightly so that you're able to remove them from the muffin tins.

Marshall explains why these are called "popovers."

Don't be rushed when eating. A lot of times if you eat fast, you don't enjoy the food and you can also choke. Buy an alarm clock if you have to get up a few minutes earlier to have time for breakfast. Or try to focus more on making time. Make sure you enjoy your food by not rushing.

Visiting an antique store or antique mall is like going to a museum. I cannot tell you how many times I have seen a child stick his or her finger into the numbers of an old rotary phone and not know how to operate it. Try taking your child to an antique shop and see how many old recipe books you can find together, or look for antique kitchen tools, like an old-fashioned reamer, Jell-O molds, or eggbeaters. Or, if you don't live near an antique mall, just visit your grandmother's house and investigate what she has hidden in her cabinets. Adding a few inexpensive historical pieces to your kitchen may help you and your children remember that the foundation of your home is your kitchen.

The Backstory on Some Handy Kitchen Tools

Gelatin or Jelly Molds

Gelatin molds were used as far back as the 1730s. During that era, gelatin molds were not the plastic or tin molds we think of today, but pierced creamware (pottery) used to shape curds and cream. Molds can also be made of wood and come in any imaginable shape and size. Some can even be made with parts that break away or create shapes.

Eggbeaters

At least one thousand patents have been issued for eggbeaters since 1856 and it seems to be the kitchen utility of extreme innovation. The earliest versions of the hand-cranked eggbeaters were made of cast iron, then made with wooden handles, and electric versions were available as early as 1911. Then in the 1930s glass-bottomed, hand-cranked, and electric mixers became popular. It simply was a jar that you screwed a lid to and attached to the lid was the mixer. The first Cuisinart!

Rolling Pins

Rolling pins are meant to flatten and shape dough and have been around for centuries. The oldest rolling pins were handcrafted of one singular piece of wood with knob endings for your hands. Later, they would be made with separate handles and ball bearings so the handles wouldn't have to slide in your hands. You can find many types and shapes of rolling pins, including a rod pin which has no handles and is tapered on either end. Glass rolling pins can be filled with cool or warm water depending on your needs. Marble, inlaid wood, carved—the list is endless in variations.

Abundance Juice

If you have an abundance of seasonal berries around, why not make your own juice concentrate from them? After rinsing the berries, put them in a pot (you can even use a mix of different types of berries) with just enough water over them that they bob. Bring to a boil and mash with a potato masher. Remove from the heat and cool a bit. Pour the berries into a coffee filter or cheese cloth. (Depending on how much you have made, you may have to do this several times. Also, remember that berry juice stains.) Gently squeeze the coffee filter, collecting the juice into a bowl. Compost or discard the remaining berry pieces from the filter and repeat as needed. Sweeten the juice with either honey or pineapple juice to taste. Now you have a bit of a juice concentrate, and you can dilute to taste with water and serve over ice, dilute with soda water and make a fruit soda, freeze in ice cube trays, or make popsicles.

Breakfast Day #4

Marshall: My Grandma Sharron had type 2 diabetes. She was one of my favorites. I know that in type 2, your body cannot absorb insulin, and with type 1, your body does not make insulin. My friend, Quinn, got type 1, and I feel really bad for him because he didn't have a choice to have this in his life. I feel pretty bad for people with type 2 because they decided to have it in their lives. Not that they choose it, but that they accept the shots and needles by basically ignoring the fact that they are being unhealthy. It makes me feel like their health is not important to them. That's one of the reasons PSM is so important to me, because I'm not gonna end up like that. I'm not going to end up this big. I'm not going to be a blueberry. I'm not! I'm not going to let myself. I'm just not. Sometimes it has kept me up at night. It's just not acceptable to me if I let it happen. It's a man-made problem and I have to put my foot down.

Alex: I remember playing marbles with an old family friend on her kitchen floor, and I have a complete visual picture of her refrigerator. Funny how you remember certain things, isn't it? I also remember she took shots in her stomach and wore really thick stockings on her feet even during the Florida summer heat. She had diabetes. Those stockings were so burned into my memory that even as a young working professional, I avoided wearing stockings or panty hose. As an adult, I now understand that people diabetes may experience a loss of feeling in their feet, and somehow the stockings help.

Now here is another story about diabetes. Last year, my sister went for an annual physical and the doctor told her she was flirting with diabetes. She got scared and really made an about-face change in her lifestyle. She started exercising and eating at home more often. Within three months, she had dropped a couple clothing sizes, her blood pressure had reduced considerably, and her blood sugar level was normal. That scare made an impression upon her the way the stockings made an impression on me. Impressions are a useful tool when you can recognize what they mean to you.

Nikki's Super-Moist Banana Bread

My girlfriend Nikki has a girl and a boy who are each a year older than my kids, and we have been friends for many years. We used to talk on the phone, inspiring each other to make new things for our families, and we would feed off each other by discussing new ideas and creative concepts. She was very much a part of our ethnic dinner parties and holidays. She moved out of town and I occasionally get to visit with her, and sometimes when I do, she gives me a tiny loaf of banana bread (which I almost always finish on my drive home). There is no way to describe how moist the bread is.

Note that there isn't any oil in this recipe, just lots of bananas.

My only change to this recipe is to use half regular and half whole-wheat flour. Also remember you may have some frozen bananas in the freezer to use.

- » 2 cups flour
- » 1 teaspoon baking soda
- » ¼ teaspoon salt
- » ¾ cup brown sugar
- » ½ cup butter, at room temperature
- » 2 eggs, beaten
- » 5 bananas, mashed

Mix together the dry ingredients: flour, baking soda, salt, and brown sugar. In a separate bowl, cream the butter, eggs, and bananas. Now gently combine the dry ingredients with the wet ingredients. "Don't go crazy," says Nikki. The batter shouldn't be overmixed. Grease a loaf pan and pour the mixture into the pan. Bake at 350°F for about 50 minutes.

>> We are still trying to add more activity to our schedule, and I suggested to Marshall that we take a trip to the gym to work out. We went and he was a bit uncomfortable. When I asked why, he couldn't really tell me. I suspected he was feeling insecure or a bit intimidated. After I explained that I thought people at the gym were cool because it was a whole roomful of people on the same mission, he relaxed.

If you choose to go out to eat, take a moment to see if the restaurant has posted a nutrition poster for the products they serve. Sometimes they can provide a brochure as well. Then decide what you want to order based on the information you learned from that. I suspect it will prevent you from frequenting those types of restaurants in the future, like it did for me.

Marshall investigates nutritional information at a local restaurant.

Diabetes

There are three major types of diabetes:

1. Type 1 diabetes is usually diagnosed in childhood. Many patients are diagnosed when they are older than age twenty. In this disease, the body makes little or no insulin. Daily injections of insulin are needed. The exact cause is unknown. Genetics, viruses, and autoimmune problems may play a role.

2. Type 2 diabetes is far more common than type 1. It makes up most of diabetes cases. It usually occurs in adulthood, but young people are increasingly being diagnosed with this disease. The pancreas does not make enough insulin to keep blood glucose levels normal, often because the body does not respond well to insulin. Many people with type 2 diabetes do not know they have it, although it is a serious condition. Type 2 diabetes is becoming more common due to increasing levels of obesity and failure to exercise.

3. Gestational diabetes is high blood glucose that develops at any time during pregnancy in a woman who does not have diabetes. Women who have gestational diabetes are at high risk of type 2 diabetes and cardiovascular disease later in life.

Breakfast Day #5

A note from Jordan: Marshall has really changed tremendously throughout this journey of Portion Size Me, and I think that's cool. I would ask Marshall, or other kids, if they are where they want to be. When they look in the mirror, do they see what they want to see? Are they happy with their self-image? And if it's not what they want to see, what do they want? And how can they reach that goal? I would ask them if they are happy. And I would ask him those questions when he is not playing video games or thinking about food. I know I don't keep my room clean, and that is self-control too, but his self-control is dangerous. Because it is so hard on your body to be overweight. You just start sweating grease and breathing heavy. There are kids in my school who are overweight, and they eat school lunches and bring snacks like candy. Every Friday, we have this greasy pizza and that is your only choice. I don't understand that. The only reason I am not big is because I don't like to eat that much and I play soccer. But there are so many overweight kids in my school. Most are not really bad, but they are big. When we had height and weight day, most of the girls asked to go into the back room to get measured. They are embarrassed already. I don't even know what a normal weight is supposed to be or look like. Everybody is judged big or skinny. I am happy with my size, but I think everyone should be happy, and overweight people need to find a way to be the size that lets them feel happy with themselves.

Alex: I know in the past that Jordan has been indignant about Marshall's plight. Portion Size Me has helped quite a bit, thanks to all the conversations we have been having and the education we have been gleaning. It also helped to pull out some old baby pictures and VHS movies. While watching the movies, I overheard Jordan say things like how cute Marshall was, and I think it has helped her to be more compassionate toward her brother.

Homemade Granola

This recipe is from my friend Julian. He is fifty and looks as if he is in his mid-thirties—probably because he grows a huge garden every year and eats very healthy. This recipe doesn't have any additional oil in it outside of the natural good-for-you oils in the nuts. Store this in individual zip-top bags and enjoy!

- » 4 cups old-fashioned whole oats (not instant)
- » ¼ cup frozen fruit juice concentrate, any flavor
- » ½ cup honey
- » 1 teaspoon cinnamon (or you can substitute with nutmeg, cloves, ginger, allspice, or cardamom)
- » ½ teaspoon almond extract (or your other favorite flavor)
- » 1 teaspoon vanilla extract
- » ½ cup chopped nuts: almonds, pecans, peanuts, or walnuts

- » ½ cup of wheat germ or flaxseed (or a combination of the two)
- » 1 cup dried fruit: cranberries, raisins, coconut, currants, golden raisins, cherries, apples, or mangos

Spray a cookie sheet (1" x 11" x 17") with low-fat cooking spray.

Spread the oats on a cookie sheet and toast them in the oven at 350°F, stirring every 2 to 3 minutes for a total of 8 to 9 minutes.

Place the juice concentrate, honey, cinnamon, almond extract, and vanilla extract in a saucepan and begin heating until it just begins to boil.

Place the toasted oats, nuts, seeds, and fruits in a large bowl. Pour the liquid honey mixture over the dry ingredients and stir until well coated. Place this mixture onto the cookie sheet.

Bake at 350°F for 30 to 45 minutes, stirring every 10 minutes, until golden brown and crunchy. Cool completely. Break into chunks the consistency that you desire.

Crepes

Crepes are thin pancakes, and you usually always have the basic ingredients to make them on hand. You can stuff them with some fresh fruit and sour cream or even just some yummy preserves.

- » 2 large eggs
- » ¾ cup milk
- » ½ cup water
- » 1 cup whole-wheat flour
- » Butter to melt in the pan
- » Fruit or preserves of your choice
- » Powdered sugar (optional)
- » Honey (optional)

Whisk the eggs, milk, water, and flour in a bowl until smooth. The batter will be watery.

Heat a nonstick pan over medium-high heat, melting a small amount of butter to coat the bottom of the pan. Pour a few tablespoons of batter onto the center of the pan (a ladle makes this easy). Rotate the pan to distribute the batter evenly around. Make the crepe as big as you can. Don't worry if it is not a perfect circle. Cook for about 1 minute. Use a spatula to turn the crepe over and cook another 1 to 2 minutes.

Place fruit or preserves on top of the crepe, and roll it up like a burrito to serve. You can sprinkle with a little powdered sugar or drizzle honey on it.

Marshall makes a variety of crepes.

Kids have great memories and are easily able to learn new things. But I think they also forget those everyday moments that build your family. Try having a family movie or picture night and bring out all the old VHS, 35mm, and other video formats. Bring out the old photo albums, or if you are like me and just have all the photos stuffed in a Rubbermaid tub, just grab a handful and work together to put them into an album.

Why did the raisin go out with the prune? Because he couldn't find a date!

Breakfast Day #6

Marshall: I know my grandpa grew up in the Depression. It was a period of time when the economy was really bad and people did not have jobs or a lot of money for food. He helped me realize that you need to enjoy food because there may come a time when you might not be able to have more. I know that is one of the reasons he is living so long. 'Cause he learned to appreciate food. He was getting food in smaller quantities and he learned to use everything. And not waste a thing. And I think that really helped him out in his lifetime and how he is living right now. I think it's because he grew up in the old days when McDonald's didn't exist, Wendy's didn't exist, Walmart didn't exist. You knew if you wanted a steak, you would either go to the butcher or go out and hunt, or, you know, slaughter a cow. I think that is very cool.

Baked Egg

I discovered this years ago when trying to figure out how to make my eggs for eggs Benedict on an Easter Sunday for about a dozen people. Grease a muffin pan with cooking spray and crack 1 or 2 eggs into the muffin hole (whether you use 1 or 2 eggs depends on the size of your muffin tin). Cook at 400°F for about 10 to 15 minutes, depending on how you want your egg cooked. Use a spoon to scoop the egg out of the tin, and serve. You can serve this on a piece of toast, on an English muffin, on a bagel, or even over a scone.

If I could figure out a way to make eggs Benedict sauce healthy, we would be eating it more than the twice a year we do. But that is what makes it special, having it on those two special days a year with a sauce in all its richness.

Alex: Marshall's grandpa grew up in Iowa during the Great Depression, and his food experiences are significantly different than Marshall's, or even Marshall's dad. Grandpa Merlin talked about one of his favorite treats as a kid. It was fresh buttermilk. This was real buttermilk, straight from the cow, not artificially cultured buttermilk, which is common today. Whenever he could, he went to his Aunt Vera's farm to enjoy a glass. Aunt Vera kept the buttermilk in a hole in the ground near the windmill that pumped water to the livestock tank. The water ran through a pipe to the hole in the ground, around the crock of buttermilk, and then through another pipe to the stock tank. Since the water was cold from being underground, it refrigerated the buttermilk. Things are so different today, but it's good to remember the past, as I think it helps one be more grounded in the current day.

Marshall enjoys doing some really old-fashioned things to entertain himself. He whittles arrows and makes spears. He has made several shields and painted them like something you might see in a movie. He built a catapult, and a while ago he had a blast with a rope and pulley. This type of self entertainment seems more "active" rather than the "passive" entertainment of television or computer games. It requires whole body involvement, physical, mental, imagination, etc. I need to work harder on encouraging him to explore more of these types of activities.

Watch Marshall use his homemade shields as a defense against water balloons!

 Day 6 Video 1

I think everybody needs to go back into the old times for one day and do everything the old-fashioned way to really appreciate and understand how easy we have it today, during modern times. Grandpa didn't start out eating all that processed stuff that could be hurting him now. What about kids today that start out eating all the fast-food stuff mostly? What are they going to be like when or if they make it to my grandpa's age?

Cholesterol is a waxy substance that's found in the fats (lipids) in your blood. While your body needs cholesterol to continue building healthy cells, having high cholesterol can increase your risk of heart disease. When you have high cholesterol, you may develop fatty deposits in your blood vessels. Eventually, these deposits make it difficult for enough blood to flow through your arteries. Your heart may not get as much oxygen-rich blood as it needs, which increases the risk of a heart attack. Decreased blood flow to your brain can cause a stroke.

High cholesterol can be inherited, but it is often preventable and treatable. A healthy diet, regular exercise, and sometimes medication can go a long way toward reducing high cholesterol.

Scones

» 1½ cups flour (I have been using half all-purpose flour and half whole-wheat flour.)
» 3 tablespoons sugar
» 2½ teaspoons baking powder
» ½ teaspoon baking soda
» ¼ teaspoon salt
» 5 tablespoons cold or frozen butter
» ⅔ cup low-fat buttermilk or regular milk
» ½ cup fruit and zest, such as raisins and dried cranberries with orange or lemon zest (optional)

In a medium bowl, mix together the flour, sugar, baking powder, baking soda, and salt. Grate the butter into the flour mixture using the large holes of a box grater, or chop the butter into little pieces and add it to the mixture. Stir in the buttermilk and any fruit or zest you are adding.

Using a fork, stir until large dough clumps form. Use your hands to press the dough against the bowl into a ball. The dough will be sticky in places, but keep working it. You can add a splash more buttermilk if the dough is not moist enough.

Place the dough onto a lightly floured surface and pat it into a 7- to 8-inch circle about ¾-inch thick. Use a sharp knife to cut it into 8 triangles; place the triangles onto a cookie sheet lined with parchment paper. Bake at 400°F for about 15 to 17 minutes, or until golden.

Breakfast Day #7

Marshall: I have learned to start looking at meals like science. I mean, before I used to just eat without any thoughts. I just ate. Now I look and say to myself, "That's a protein, and that's calcium." I know the nutritional value of the food I am looking at. I am starting to look at food as nourishment, not emotional eating. If you're eating to feed your body, then you're going to be just fine.

Roasted Acorn Squash with Cinnamon

Why not start your day out with squash? It's rich in vitamins and fiber. You may consider prepping this dish the night before (or asking your child to prepare it the night before), as the cook time is a little longer than a normal breakfast. But once you stick it in the oven, you are done with it.

- » 1 acorn squash
- » A drizzle of real maple syrup
- » 2 pinches cinnamon

Microwave the acorn squash for four to five minutes and then cut it into quarters, scooping out and discarding the seeds. Place the wedges on foil in a glass baking dish. Evenly cover with the syrup and cinnamon, and wrap solidly in aluminum. Add about ½ inch water to the baking dish, around the foil. Now you can put the dish in the fridge until the morning, or you can go ahead and bake at 400°F for about 40 minutes.

Alex: Why can we not have a regular burrito for breakfast? It has to be a breakfast burrito. A piece of chocolate after dinner is dessert, but any other time, it's a snack or just wrong to have. I am not sure how this food prejudice of eating certain things at certain times began. But let's break through those barriers. Both my kids love sugar snap peas and we regularly have them in the freezer to use for a dinner. Why can we not have them for breakfast? "They are only meant for dinner," the kids argue with me. Food prejudice! It limits your options, and quite frankly, all this self-education I am doing here with PSM shows me how nutritionally incomplete some meals are, especially breakfasts on the go.

> My aunt taught me to use a zip-top bag to squeeze out the deviled egg mixture back into the egg whites to make deviled eggs. You just fill the bag with your mixture, cut a small bit of the corner off the bag, and then you squeeze the stuff through the hole. It works pretty nice!

Thanks to our world getting smaller new healthy options are cropping up all the time at your local store. Keep your eyes open to discover new delights like chia seeds, cupuacu, goji berries, and dandelion greens. I'm not saying you have to live at a health-food store. What I am saying is that...well...that breakfasts are very difficult for me as a mom and I will open every door possible to expand our repertoire to make that job easier in a healthy way.

Squash

Squashes are the fruits of various members of the gourd family, and they are native to the Western Hemisphere. There is evidence of squash being eaten in Mexico as far back as 5,500 BCE and in South America over 2,000 years ago.

Squashes vary widely in size, shape, and color. Generally, they're divided into two categories: summer squash and winter squash. Summer squashes have thin, edible skins and soft seeds. The tender flesh has a high water content and a mild flavor, and they don't require long cooking. The most widely available varieties of summer squashes are crookneck, pattypan, and zucchini. Summer squashes are best from early through late summer, although some varieties are available year-round in certain regions. Select the smaller specimens with bright-colored skin free of spots and bruises. Summer squash is very perishable and should be refrigerated in a plastic bag for no more than five days. It can be prepared by a variety of methods, including steaming, baking, sautéing, and deep-frying. Summer squash is high in vitamins A and C as well as niacin.

Winter squashes have hard, thick skins and seeds. The deep yellow to orange flesh is firmer than that of summer squash and therefore requires longer cooking. Winter squash varieties include acorn, buttercup, butternut, hubbard, spaghetti, and turban. Though most varieties are available year-round, winter squash is best from early fall through the winter. Choose squashes that are heavy for their size and have a hard, deep-colored rind free of blemishes or moldy spots. The hard skin of a winter squash protects the flesh and allows it to be stored longer than a summer squash. It does not require refrigeration and can be kept in a cool, dark place for a month or more, depending on the variety. Once the seeds are removed, winter squashes can be baked, steamed, or simmered. They're a good source of iron, riboflavin, and vitamin A.

Deviled Eggs

» Eggs (however many you want to make)
» Celery, minced
» Onion, minced
» Spinach, minced
» Bacon or turkey bacon, finely chopped
» Lots of minced garlic
» A bit of light mayo, just enough to get things mixed together
» A dash of Worcestershire sauce
» Salt and pepper
» Fresh cilantro, minced

Hard-boil the eggs. Once they have cooled, peel and slice them in half. Scoop the yolks into a bowl and add the rest of the ingredients, through salt and pepper. Mash and blend all the ingredients together, adding more light mayo if you want a creamier texture. (I personally like my egg filling chunky to contrast with the creamy bite of the egg white.) Spoon the mixture into each little egg-white half and garnish with the cilantro.

Breakfast Day #8

Marshall: I think it's a great idea for my mom to encourage parents to get into the kitchen and for me to encourage kids to talk to their parents about getting in the kitchen and helping out. Why not? It's safe, fun, and healthy. And it makes you happy to be with your family. And when you're an adult you will know how to cook for yourself.

Ambrosia

I believe this is a throwback to the 1950s It's a little heavy in the calorie department, and it does use marshmallows, which are processed, but remember: success comes from eating in moderation and not completely depriving yourself of treats. It's about eating comforting meals every day, exploring new things, and cooking them together in the kitchen with the family.

» 1 large can fruit cocktail, drained (Check the ingredients on the can to ensure it's not too high in fat or artificial ingredients.)
» 1 large can mandarin oranges, drained (Make sure the can doesn't contain added sugar.)
» 1 banana, sliced
» 2 handfuls mini marshmallows
» 1 handful chopped walnuts
» ½ handful coconut flakes
» 1 small container low-fat sour cream
» A drizzle of agave nectar or honey

Mix all the ingredients together in a large bowl and chill. The coconut really adds sweetness to the dish. Serve!

Alex: There are definite advantages to rising earlier in the morning. I am not particularly a morning glory, but awaking at 6 a.m. would fit my internal clock perfectly. That is what time I get the kids up for school as well. But with dogs needing to be walked and a dire need for a cup in coffee in the morning, my alarm is set at 5:30. Sometimes I do hit the snooze button, and just having ten minutes to get those things done before the morning chaos starts is helpful. Truthfully, a routine is convenience unto itself, and if you can give yourself just a few more minutes in the morning to work into a routine, the whole house may be happier.

In my eyes I think of obesity and bad foods as a battle. On one side is good food and fitness; on the other side is bad food and obesity. And right now my feelings are that America as a country is too obese. The obesity and bad foods are winning. The obesity rate in America is like 20 percent. That means 1 in every 5 people is obese. So many people are trying to stop this, and that will happen. I hope it happens soon.

PORTION SIZE ME

I was talking to my husband about breakfast time and how the options for breakfast have always felt limited. He asked me when I started thinking, as in mentally planning, for breakfast. My answer: at breakfast, of course. Hmmm. His suggestion was to start thinking about it at dinner the night before. I like that idea, so I am passing it on to you.

Warm Milk

I always enjoy a cup of coffee or two in the morning. Sometimes the kids like to have something warm in the morning as well. They like teas, chais, and sometimes just warm milk. You can add a natural sweetener, like honey, if needed. Add a squeeze of lemon, lime, or orange to the hot tea. Or even add a pinch of cinnamon to the warm milk. It just feels cozy having a warm drink in the morning and these are pretty good options that the kids can make themselves.

In Greek mythology, ambrosia was the honey-flavored food eaten by the gods that allowed them to remain immortal. With the ambrosia, they often drank a honey-flavored drink called nectar. According to legend, each day doves brought ambrosia to Zeus, the king of the gods, to distribute among the other deities. Humans who ate ambrosia grew faster, stronger, and more beautiful, all qualities that were considered divine. Eating ambrosia also made humans immortal. In one Greek myth, a son of Zeus's named Tantalus was punished for crimes that included stealing ambrosia from heaven and giving it to humans.

Beekeeper, Julian Youngblood: I started beekeeping by winning a lottery from North Carolina State University. They had over 2,000 entries for just 250 winners. Each winner got two hives, one with Russian bees and one with Italian bees. Each winner had to agree to help study the effects of Varroa mites on each hive and report back to the university. Well, I was hooked and have had bees for five years now. Bees are extremely important to our food supply. Many crops *must* be pollinated by bees! Foods like almonds, cucumbers, melons, berries, apples, and cocoa can't bear fruit without the bees. Luckily for us, honey is the by-product of this pollination! Honey has been used by humans for millennia. Cave drawings in Spain from six thousand years ago show honey being gathered, and honey has been found in Egyptian tombs. Because honey never goes bad, three-thousand-year-old honey is still safe to eat! Honey has awesome antibacterial properties and can even be used to heal cuts and sores. Honey has sixty calories per tablespoon of all-natural sweetness! There are no chemicals or processing involved. So when someone calls you "honey," it's a pretty big compliment!

Breakfast Day #9

Marshall: Rome wasn't built in a day, so don't immediately think you're going to go from one thousand pounds to three pounds, you know. It takes time—a lot of time and work. And you have to be willing to dish that out; you have to be willing to work hard. Be patient. I know a lot of people quit after so long because they think, "Oh no, there aren't enough results." You're not going to get immediate results except for your energy and how you feel.

Immediately, you will feel refreshed and feel fine. That's good. Let that carry you until your body starts to show results too. My aunt spoke earlier about having a mind-set to eat right. She is right, you have to have a mind-set to build Rome and build your body.

waldorf salad

» Equal amounts of diced celery and firm, red apples with skin left on
» Half as much chopped walnuts and sliced seedless grapes or raisins
» Couple spoonfuls of light mayonnaise
» To sweeten the flavor a bit you can add honey or agave nectar. To make it tangier, add a squeeze of lemon juice. You can really make it to fit your taste.

Mix all the ingredients. You want the salad to be lightly coated in the mayo, not sopping wet.

Traditionally, this is served over lettuce, but why not try wrapping it in lettuce? This salad can be made anytime and kept easily in the fridge to serve on busy mornings.

Alex: Have you ever heard of a "cold car start?" It's when you start your car in the morning and it lags, sputters, coughs, and takes a few seconds to start humming. You cannot really drive it until it is warmed up and all the parts and functions are working together in harmony. That's a good analogy for warming up your body before exercise too. Start slow and give yourself a few minutes to get all the joints, muscles, and tendons working together.

> Don't listen to your own excuses. Pretend that someone else said them and then help that pretend other person find a solution.

Do you have a good neighbor friend? Or work colleague? Someone you have a close relationship with and who lives or works near you? Why not exchange salads? One day one person can make enough for two families, and the next day the other can make enough for all. This would free up some time and energy used in the mornings. You don't have to do it every day of the week, perhaps every Monday and Friday!

There are multiple reasons for stretching, either to prepare for more strenuous exercise or just to increase your flexibility and keep your muscles and joints healthy. We've always been taught to stretch before exercise; however, more recently, emphasis has been placed on getting the body slightly "warmed up" and then doing some light stretching to prepare the muscles for the more vigorous activity.

Stretching is not for athletes only. More and more these days, large companies are learning the benefits of keeping their employees healthier in multiple ways. They find that the healthier the employees are, the more productive they are. Large manufacturing companies have begun incorporating stretching into part of the workday. Even though this takes what would normally be valuable time away from labor, corporations have found that productivity ultimately increases as a result of the investment in keeping their employees' bodies limber. Additionally, work-related injuries are decreased through both stretching and having physically fit associates. This decrease in harm for the employee and decrease in "lost time" for the employer is a win-win for everyone.

Regardless of when you choose to stretch or for which reason, there is no doubt that stretching increases blood flow to the tissues, increases the tensile strength of tissue, promotes balance and flexibility, and minimizes tension—all contributing to an alert but relaxed readiness for the day. That is why many people choose yoga, Tai Chi, or Pilates as one of their primary modes of feeling good and contributing to their overall wellness.
—Leslie Byrne, RN, MSN, NP-C

Fruit Cubes

Honestly, this idea came up with a couple of friends of mine to flavor our Friday night margaritas. We used watermelon ice cubes for the margaritas, and it was very refreshing, but any fresh or leftover fruit will do. Just blend it in a blender and pour the liquid into ice cube trays. Once frozen, you can keep the ice cubes in a zip-top bag for a long period of time. You can use the fruit cubes to flavor water, tea, soda water (to make a fruit soda), or of course, your margarita.

Watch Marshall prepare watermelon ice cubes.

Day 9
Video 1

Mayonnaise is an emulsion, which is a mixture of two liquids that normally can't be combined. Combining oil and water is the classic example. By slowly adding one ingredient to another while mixing very rapidly, it appears if they can be mixed. However, the two liquids would quickly separate again if an emulsifier was not added. Emulsifiers are a connection between the two liquids and serve to stabilize the mixture. Eggs and gelatin are among the foods that contain emulsifiers. In mayonnaise, the emulsifier is egg yolk, which contains lecithin, a fat emulsifier.

Breakfast Day #10

Marshall: Enjoy the little things! What that means to me is to say if, for example, I can only have a Twinkie once a month, I should slow down and enjoy it. If I slow down and enjoy that Twinkie, spacing eating it out and not just eating it in one bite, I get more from it than just wolfing it down. You can take smaller bites of it. Cut it in half, eat half now and the other half a few minutes later. What I have noticed is, most people just chew their food and swallow it. It's kinda like giving my dog a cookie treat: he doesn't even taste it. Boom, it's gone. You don't get the whole flavor when you wolf it down. If I'm having beef jerky, for example, what I like to do is put the jerky in my mouth, suck on it a bit, then chew on it and really take my time. That gives you the whole flavor. So enjoy the little things, like these Twinkie and beef jerky examples. Of course, I don't really mean to eat a Twinkie; that's just my example. Whatever special treat you get, if it's for a holiday or not, take your time and appreciate it.

Alex: One of the biggest things I have learned through this PSM process is to actually consider the nutritional value of what we put into our bodies. That is not even a specific goal, but a by-product of choosing to eat real foods. Of course, fruits and vegetables have always been a delicious and colorful contribution to my personal diet. But I have always viewed my diet as a requirement or deserved satisfaction and not a nutritional resource. It really is an outlook shift that has occurred within me, and I hope within my family members.

Fitness as well has been a new inspiration to me, thanks to PSM. For example, I play tennis and walk and jog. So I consider myself in pretty good cardiovascular shape. But now that we are playing more, shooting hoops, kayaking, and riding bikes, I realize that there is a lot more to the world of fitness: endurance, stamina, and drive. Couple that with the energy kids have and the fact that my body is a little tiny bit older than their bodies; my eyes have been opened to paying attention to my own physical health.

Ceviche

Ceviche is made with raw fish that is essentially cooked in fresh citrus juices. The variations of ceviche are limitless, from the types of seafood (fish, shrimp, crab, or conch) to the marinade (lemon, lime, or grapefruit juice) to the additional ingredients (onion, nuts, seaweed, chiles). Ceviche is a staple dish in many places.

Although my kids will eat sushi with cooked fish, I didn't think raw fish would go over particularly well with them. And I didn't want to be responsible for accidentally making them ill if I messed up, so we used cooked seafood. We make this ceviche for a special brunch rather than a school day breakfast. Even though this recipe has a lot of ingredients, a child can easily put it together.

- » 1 bag precooked, peeled, deveined shrimp, chopped
- » 1 red onion, minced
- » ½ bunch fresh cilantro, chopped
- » 2 large tomatoes
- » 1 serrano chile pepper, seeded and minced
- » ½ cucumber or jicama, peeled and diced
- » Dash salt
- » Dash hot sauce
- » Dash oregano
- » 1 tablespoon olive oil
- » Juice of 2 large limes
- » Juice of 2 large lemons

Place the shrimp, onion, cilantro, tomatoes, chiles, cucumber, salt, hot sauce, oregano, and olive oil in a glass bowl. Cover with the lime and lemon juice. Let sit for an hour, then stir. Let sit for at least another hour.

This tasty dish can be eaten with crackers, tortilla chips, and bread. But my fave is to pull out a wine glass and serve it that way. The kids feel special when treated with the finer items in the house.

Have you smelled your food lately? I don't mean to see if it's gone bad. But to see if you know what's in it, especially if it is something new like this ceviche. I know, I am just starting to take that step, and I wondered if you do it too.

Having grown up in San Fran and Florida, seafood has always been a part of my diet. And any time I pulled in my crab trap off of Elephant Rock to bring home Dungeness crab for dinner, it never smelled. Not even like the bay water. Seafood, if fresh, should never smell. Even if you walk into a fresh seafood market, if the food really is fresh, the market should never smell or be filled with cleaning-product odors. Trust your nose: it knows!

Acids, like lemon juice used in ceviche, are natural tenderizers that break down connective tissues and cell walls in food.

Vegetable Juice

Since we are talking about brunch, versus breakfast at its usual time, that to me means a more lingering and enjoyable meal. One that is savored and includes much conversation and respectful debate between loved ones. So we can pair our delightful ceviche with something delicious and healthy to drink. Start with a tomato-based product like plain tomato juice or a low sodium V8 juice in a cocktail shaker or use a pitcher and spoon. Then add a bit of the following to taste:

- » Cracked pepper
- » Worcestershire sauce
- » Lemon juice

Then to really go over the top on this drink, add any or all of the following (in order of my favorites):

- » Celery salt
- » Pick-A-Pepper Sauce
- » Fresh (or creamed) horseradish
- » Tabasco sauce
- » Garlic salt

Serve over ice with a celery stalk in the glass.

There is one other ingredient you can add to the adult glasses if you wish!

Track

Your Journey!

A Note from Jordan:
If I had a friend who needed more exercise, I wouldn't tell him that. I would just invite him to do something without him knowing it. I would just say, "Hey, do you want to go pass the soccer ball?" or something like that. It's better to have fun than to make things work all the time, anyway.

Track

Your Journey!

Ten Days
of Lunches

Lunch Day #1

satay skewers

This is an Indonesian hot dish, but it can be served equally well in a lunch box. It can be made the night before while you're preparing the main dinner, or if you do advance prep work on the weekend to get ready for the upcoming week, you can put this together then. Make a dozen or so of these beauties and everyone can have them for lunch. Make sure, however, that you remove the bamboo skewer if you are going to send this to school, as the skewers may be frowned upon these days by school administrators.

- » 2 tablespoons natural peanut butter
- » ½ cup soy sauce
- » 2 squeezes lime juice
- » 1 tablespoon brown sugar
- » Lots of minced garlic
- » Pinch cumin
- » Salt and pepper
- » Lean beef or chicken cut into 2-inch strips

Mix the peanut butter, soy sauce, lime juice, brown sugar, garlic, cumin, and salt and pepper in a large bowl. Add the meat to the marinade and place in the fridge for a minimum of a half an hour. Soak the bamboo skewers in water while the meat marinates.

You can cook these on the grill outside or under the oven broiler. Cook thoroughly.

When you eat these at a restaurant, they usually serve additional peanut sauce, but we choose not to and just enjoy the light peanut flavor on the meat itself.

Marshall: PSM is all about stopping and standing up for yourself. The greasy hamburger and French fries are the mean guys. If you never stand up for yourself, like I am, you are going to get beat up. Your body will get beat up. Not literally like a black and blue punch but in an unhealthy way you're going to get beat up. I am standing up for you guys. I want to help you guys out as well as helping myself out with my life and family. If you never stand up for yourself, then the mean guy will be even worse, and worse and worse. But if you stand up for yourself and you fight back by exercising and having good allies like good fruit and healthy foods and all that stuff, then you're gonna end up on one of those TV shows about the world's fittest man, or world's fittest woman, or world's fittest kid. Kids who could run a mile or eight miles without having to stop. You will be fit if you stand up for yourself. Right now I am standing up for myself and for everyone else who is having a hard time. And I am encouraging you to stand up for yourself so we can say no to that mean guy, those greasy hamburgers and stuff.

Alex: Working together in the kitchen has really opened my eyes to how much this experience is teaching Marshall. He is learning about cause and effect in a whole new way, beyond the fundamental understanding that water does boil over and make a mess. He is learning how to predict the outcome of a kitchen adventure, whether good or bad. Although he has not had a knife accident yet, he is acutely aware that it is a real possibility and he must be quite diligent in being slow and paying attention so as not to need a Band-Aid.

My mom has commented to me a few times saying, "Wow! You're looking slimmer," or "You're looking like you're getting a little bit faster!" That makes me smile.

We found another inexpensive and fun exercise that can also be done indoors. Boxing. I picked up one pair of gloves and a set of hitting pads for another person to wear on his or her hands. Marshall and I take turns, and it's quite fun and tiring.

Garbanzo Snacks

"Garbanzo": what a fun word to say! Jordan likes to munch on these, and they are easy and healthy. You can make them spicier or milder, to your taste. This is Jordan's recipe.

- » 2 cans garbanzo beans, drained and dried on a paper towel
- » Powdered beef boullion
- » Salt and pepper
- » Garlic powder
- » Ground red pepper
- » Cumin
- » Dried basil
- » Dried rosemary

Place the garbanzo beans in a bowl and mix with the remaining ingredients. Place the beans on a cookie sheet. Roast at 350°F for about 25 minutes, and then gently toss the beans in the pan to recoat them with seasoning mixture. Cool and enjoy. Make sure you seal leftovers in an airtight container, as they will get stale quickly.

Food Allergies

An estimated 3.9 percent of children under the age of eighteen and 2 percent of adults have food allergies. Though reasons for this are poorly understood, the prevalence of food allergies and associated anaphylaxes appears to be on the rise. There are eight foods that account for 90 percent of all food-allergy reactions: cow's milk, egg, peanut, tree nuts (for example, walnuts, pecans, almonds, and cashews), fish, shellfish, soybeans, and wheat.

Symptoms of a food-allergy reaction can be sudden and severe, and they commonly include one or more of the following:

hives	difficulty breathing	coughing or wheezing
tingling in the mouth	abdominal cramps	loss of consciousness
swelling of the tongue and throat	vomiting or diarrhea	dizziness
	eczema or rash	

Chickpeas (also called garbanzo beans) are larger than the average pea and are tan or buff-colored. These legumes have a firm texture and a mild nutlike flavor. They are used in dishes extensively in the Mediterranean region, India, and the Middle East, but they have also found their way into Mexican and U.S. cuisine. They are low in saturated fat, very low in cholesterol and sodium, and a good source of dietary fiber and protein.

Lunch Day #2

Marshall: *It's really hard to make changes at school. You really don't have a choice of what to eat. You can eat this, this, and this with THIS, or you can eat this, this, and this with THAT. They usually have two main dishes and two sides. Sometimes they have a hamburger with so much cheese on it, you might as well call it a grilled cheese. Sometimes they serve green beans or corn with butter on them as a side! The macaroni and cheese is like paste. I don't think there are any noodles in it. They have ice cream daily and Rice Krispies treats. They also serve flavored milks and juice. On the lunch menu they advertise whole-grain buns but I think they are white wheat buns, not actual whole grains. It's just not appetizing.*

Wonder Bread was the United States' first sliced bread, and it was the first bread company to enrich its breads when the government supported a move to do so. But with our current diets so loaded with carbs—and with many bread options to choose from with various ingredients added to increase the shelf life, enhance flavors, and compete against other brands—it's important to take a moment and decide if you even want bread for something like a sandwich. Lettuce leaves are a crispy alternative to bread. But if you choose to use bread, make sure you read and understand the ingredients.

Watch Marshall explore bread at the grocery store, where he discovers that some contain high-fructose corn syrup and other ingredients he cannot even pronounce.

Alex: For most parents, it's hard to get the kids going on a school morning, and you certainly don't want to add to that by making them make their own lunches—unless of course, you are that rare breed who are early birds and are completely organized. But one neat thing about all this cooking we are doing together is the many multitasking lessons kids are learning. Consider making lunch together the night before while you're making dinner. Your children *will* be able to walk and chew gum at the same time as adults, thanks to all your patience and efforts now.

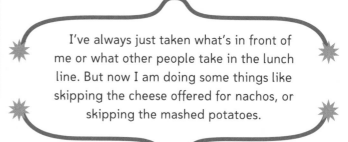

I've always just taken what's in front of me or what other people take in the lunch line. But now I am doing some things like skipping the cheese offered for nachos, or skipping the mashed potatoes.

What is cooking to you? Is it a chore? Is it fun? Is it a necessity? What do you want it to be?

Are You Fortified or Enriched?

In the early 1920s, medical and scientific studies in the United States and Europe showed that the addition of iodine to the diet aids in the prevention of common diseases such as goiter. Various agencies soon embarked on a campaign of education, promoting the addition of iodine to ordinary table salt. This is one of the first examples of fortification of a food. Fortified foods have had nutrients added to them in order to provide additional benefits over what they naturally contain.

Today, we see a host of food products that are fortified to provide nutritional benefit. From vitamin D–fortified milk to bread fortified with folic acid, they are all around us.

In addition to fortification, some foods are "enriched." The difference between fortified and enriched foods is quite simple. While fortified foods have had nutrients added that they originally did not contain, enriched foods have nutrients added to them that they originally contained, but that were lost when the food was processed, stored, or handled. Enriched flour is flour that has had vitamin B added after processing. The fortification and enrichment of foods has expanded greatly over the years. Items added include not only vitamins but also minerals and proteins.

Lunch Rolls

Day 2 — Video 2

Today we made ham and cucumber rolls with a small dab of light ranch dressing. We included grapes, a peach, and some raw almonds in the lunch. You really have several choices in making these lunch rolls. You can either roll thinly sliced ham around a few match-stick sized pieces of cucumber, or you can use a potato peeler and make thin slices of cucumber and wrap that around a small piece of ham. Also, at some unique kitchen supply stores you can find various implements that peel cucumbers and other veggies into different shapes. Many of these tools are fun and safe for children to use. This is light and fresh and easy for Marshall, or any kid, to make on his own.

Check out what Marshall's lunch box looked like.

Believed to have originated in either India or Thailand, the cucumber has been cultivated for thousands of years. Cucumbers are usually eaten raw, and the smaller cucumber varieties are used for pickles. As a cucumber matures, the seeds grow larger and more bitter. Therefore, the seeds of an older cucumber should be removed before it's used. The more expensive English (or hothouse) cucumber can grow up to two feet long and is virtually seedless. Cucumbers are available year-round, with the peak crop from May to August. Choose firm fruit with smooth, brightly colored skins; avoid those that are shriveled or that contain soft spots. Store whole cucumbers, unwashed, in a plastic bag in the refrigerator up to ten days. Wash thoroughly just before using. Cut cucumbers can be refrigerated, tightly wrapped, for up to five days.

Lunch Day #3

Marshall: We went to Raven Rock State Park the other day, and I am literally sore. I can pick up my leg and feel huge muscles sore. And I will tell you one thing: that is awesome to feel even though it hurts. The first few times you feel like gosh, just get the pain out, but then you will want to go do some more. When you're sore like that, that means you're building muscle. We did a lot of swimming and climbing and there are a million stairs to get down to the river, so that means you have to climb them to get back to the car.

Check out Marshall during his day at Raven Rock.

Day 3 Videos 1-2

Turkey Green Sandwich

Day 3 Video 3

Today we made turkey sandwiches on whole-wheat bread. We added lots of green sprouts, sugar snap peas, and spinach with a wasabi mayo. We skipped the cheese and did not add tomatoes, as they can sometimes make the bread soggy. Sprouts are really very fresh and add a nice crunch and texture to the sandwich. Another idea is to send along a slice of fresh lime in the lunch box. Both my kids really enjoy fresh lime squeezed on greens, rice, the tortilla soup, beef, corn on the cob and much more. It must be something about the tartness or the freshness that adds value to whatever you are spritzing. This sandwich can also be made open faced to reduce the amount of bread and encourage the eating of more greens. Add an orange and a rice pudding cup, and you have a super lunch.

Watch Marshall talk about the contents of today's lunch.

Alex: If you were to ask me if I considered our family to be an outdoors-type family, I would say yes. We don't go camping, as we do like our creature comforts, but as soon as the kids had their feet on the ground, I was taking them to creeks, ponds, lakes, and rivers. We have walked about every trail in our county, ridden our bikes on our greenways, and now are exploring the waters via kayak and canoe. I really love spending this time with the kids. They are with us (in the home) for such a short period of time, so I really want to work harder to not work against them but to work with them and have us all appreciate our times together.

We played with a medicine ball the other day, which is a heavy leather ball used in a gym. Wow. Wow. It was fun 'cause I almost knocked my mother over, but it really made you breathe hard too. Who knew throwing a ball could do that?

This may seem corny, but it will work with a youngster. You can try this next time you are making a sandwich or a wrap and they want cheese. Get out a large cookie cutter, say one that is a heart shape, and have them press the cutter into the cheese. Now have them put the one with the heart on their portion, and you take the remainder, with the heart cut out. Now you each have roughly only half a slice of cheese.

Leftovers from breakfast are perfect to add to a lunch. Today we added scones. Easy to carry; easy to snack on. We did have bread with our sandwich and scones are more carbs, but this was a picnic lunch and we knew we would be out for many hours playing hard.

Citrus plants are evergreen trees or shrubs that produce fruit such as limes, oranges, grapefruits, lemons, kumquats, and more. Christopher Columbus brought oranges to the New World, and citrus was often prized as a delicacy. Most citrus fruits are peeled and the rinds are discarded, but if you finely grate the rind, you'll have zest, which you can mix into foods to flavor them.

A **carbohydrate** is a broad category of sugars, starches, and fibers that the body converts to glucose (sugar), your body's primary source of energy. There are two categories of carbohydrates, simple and complex. The body absorbs simple carbohydrates, including sugars, fruits, and vegetables, very quickly. Complex carbohydrates take longer to digest and provide more nutrients and long-term energy; they can be found in such things as whole grains and legumes (beans).

What is an astronaut's favorite sandwich? Launch meat!

Lunch Day #4

Marshall: *It's a really good idea to explore and get new things, because kids with packed lunches are getting really tired of PB&J* and juice boxes. Kids: you should try exploring on the Internet for any farms in your area. Talk to your parents about going to the farm and getting some of the fresh crops. In my area, we have the option of strawberry farms to go pick from. It's a good way to support local farmers too. Use those special foods you get once in a while to spice up your lunch boxes. How about a strawberry and peanut butter sandwich?

Alex: Although we live within the city limits, it feels very rural here. There are remnants of old farm equipment, barns, and chicken coops on our property and our neighbors' properties. So it seemed quite natural to accept little chicks given to my daughter, Jordan, to raise for her 4-H club. After building a chicken coop, showing our chickens at the county and state fairs, utilizing them in school science fair projects (no harm came to any little peep), and developing friendships with the cluckers, the city in which we reside found out and said "out" with them. It was against the city ordinance to have them. We fought and had the ordinance changed, and thankfully we got our chicks back legally, thanks in part to many progressive folks who paved the path. Anyway, you would be surprised by how many urban municipalities do allow laying hens and even bees. For example the tops of some of Manhattan's tallest buildings are homes to rooftop gardens, honeybees, and laying hens. Right there in the city. You might consider looking into your city ordinance to see what is allowed so that you can enjoy healthy food and a fun hobby.

Pickled Eggs

Pickled eggs are great for lunches, picnics, snacks, salads, or sandwiches. They are easy to make, with a lot of different ways to be creative with them. We keep ours very simple.

Hard-boil and peel the eggs. Place them in a glass container, cover with white vinegar, and seal the lid tightly. Place the jar in the fridge, and enjoy them anytime. The longer they sit, the stronger they will taste.

Options: You can make them sweeter by adding a few whole cloves and a dash of cinnamon. Or you can make them spicy by adding a few drops of Tabasco sauce or some freshly cracked pepper. You can reuse pickle juice and the pickle jar and just put the eggs in it. I have wanted to add a few springs of rosemary to a batch, but I haven't gotten around to it yet.

Cooking and helping my mom gives me something to do in my boredom time. And it's been fun to do some things I have never done before like chopping cilantro, making my own Mulligan stew, and rolling my own sushi. This is expanding our horizons.

I do believe extensive research has been done by scientists and many a mother to figure out how to peel a hardboiled egg. Normally it's easy, but sometimes the shell takes the egg white away with it. I am going to explain with complete confidence what you have to do to avoid this. Don't try to peel fresh eggs! Yup, the eggs you receive from the store have been around for a few weeks, enough time for air to get in between the shell and the membrane, making them easy to peel. Fresh eggs can be difficult to peel because the membranes are still clinging to the shell. You can try some old wives' tale tricks, such as plunging the eggs in ice-cold water. That may help, but the best remedy is to write the date two weeks in the future on your carton of fresh eggs and let them sit until that time.

Vinegar

I am sure that the people who discovered that grape juice, when left to ferment, turns into wine were very happy about their discovery (although probably a bit sad the next morning!). This wine (or other fermented liquid such as beer or cider) will continue to change if left to the natural effects of bacterial activity. The eventual outcome is a weak solution of acetic acid, which we call vinegar.

The preservative powers of vinegar have been very popular over the years, largely due to its ease of use. Simply immerse food in a jar of vinegar and seal it tightly. Then, when you need it, open and enjoy. As much as seven thousand years ago, ancient civilizations used it to preserve foods for later use. In the 1800s, the British military used vinegar not only to preserve their sea stores, but also to wash down the decks of their ships. During World War I, vinegar was used not only as a food preservative, but also a medical treatment for soldiers wounded on the battlefield.

The exquisite Italian balsamic vinegar, made from white Trebbiano grape juice, gets its dark color and pungent sweetness from aging in barrels—of various woods and in graduating size—over a period of years. You can also have herb vinegars, fruit vinegars, and the sweet rice vinegar so widely used in Asian cooking.

Lunches can be a challenge to not be boring, so today we went to a store out of town to explore options not readily available to us. It was fun to get a different perspective, and we found things like:

» Natural apple juice in the perfect lunch-size container
» All-real fruit strips that tasted just like Fruit Roll-Ups
» Dried fruits
» Natural strawberry licorice
» 100 percent real puddings

So if your town does not have a unique place to go, consider searching for one the next time you leave town to go to a mall or on vacation. You can bring a bag full of unique things home with you to include in lunches every once in a while.

Marshall explores a new grocery store to get ideas for future lunches.

Long before the days of refrigeration, the ancient Chinese stored eggs up to several years by burying them in a variety of mixtures such as salt and wet clay; cooked rice, salt, and lime; or salt and wood ashes. Today, eggs preserved in this manner are enjoyed in China as a delicacy and are called century eggs or thousand year eggs, the latter taking about one hundred days to reach its full rotten potency.

Lunch Day #5

Marshall: My mom is changing. She is not just deciding on things at the last minute. She is no longer creating at the last minute. She plans ahead which helps us in not going to fast food. She is now more like, "Marshall, will you help me?" or she asks me what I want. We plan more now in advance and I think it is a great help that I am doing this not only to my mom but for the whole household. My dad is very supportive and talks to me about what Iraqis eat since he is over there right now. I can help cook and clean meats and stuff like that. Now I can actually pitch in with all the cooking and cleaning. I know that sounds like girly stuff but really it's not. It's really cool.

From Marshall's dad, Dan: When Marshall started PSM I was serving in Iraq. Marshall sounded excited about the idea and as time went on his excitement grew. I still remember him telling me his accomplishments, recipes, and weight losses with the different things he was experimenting with as he developed PSM into a full program. The energy he showed in his videos and the focus he had on PSM made me the proudest Dad around! At first I was a bit skeptical about his ability to stick to the program. But the videos showed that not only was he determined to stick to it, but the results were there as well. As I watched the videos, I saw him truly happy about what he was doing. Marshall's excitement led me to reevaluate my lifestyle while deployed. I was in an area that was not conducive to running outside, so I found a treadmill and got back into exercising daily. I also started watching more closely what I ate and cut out a lot of the extras.

Marshall's initial videos on YouTube were fun to watch and I looked forward each morning to checking for new ones. When my wife told me CNN had contacted her and wanted to interview Marshall, I was a bit concerned that Marshall might not do well in the interview. After all, he was only ten years old. After the first interview, my concerns were removed as I watched Marshall step up and respond in a clear and mature manner. He showed me that not only was he taking the PSM program seriously, but that he serious about the results he wanted. I spent the next week downloading and showing the CNN interview and YouTube videos to anyone who walked within 10 feet of my computer.

Gnocchi

Gnocchi is an Italian dumpling made from potatoes, sweet potatoes, or sometimes flour. You can purchase them in a package in the noodle department of a grocery store. Fancier stores have sweet potato gnocchi, which is our favorite and does not taste like sweet potatoes. You just quickly boil these little gems or bake them with a little olive oil and salt and pepper. You can get quite creative with them by adding fresh sauces, diced vegetables, or even nuts. When we boil ours, I add a little tomato sauce and Asiago cheese, then keep it hot in a thermos appropriate for school.

Marshall prepares a pot of gnocchi for lunch.

> I am feeling so improved, but I do need to make a few more adjustments on how much exercise I get.

My sister, Pilar, and I used to make fairy houses out of a deck of cards when we were kids. It took a lot of time and patience stacking the cards on end to make walls, and sometimes we made the houses several stories high. Marshall has always complained that he has nothing to do, so I thought of my old card game with my sister. It's not a real physical activity, but it does get us away from the TV.

Understanding Food Dates

Sell-by date: Refers to the last day a retailer can display a product for sale; typically a food is safe to eat for ten days after the sell-by date if refrigerated properly.

Use-by date: Refers to the last day a product will maintain its optimum freshness, flavor, and texture. Beyond this date, the product begins to deteriorate, although it is still edible.

Expiration date: Means what it says—if you haven't used a product by this date, toss it.

Dried fruit is fruit where the majority of the water content is removed either naturally, through sun drying, or through the use of a dehydrator. Half of all the dried fruits sold today are raisins, followed by dates and prunes. Some fruits, such as cranberries, blueberries, and cherries, are infused with a sweetener prior to drying.

Homemade Trail Mix

Day 5 Video 2

When I was growing up, I was invited to go backpacking through the Sierra Mountains for five days. The experience was so wonderful, I cannot even articulate it. One part that made an impression upon me was making homemade trail mix beforehand. There was something about having all those separate ingredients, which seemed to me like things that could not possibly fit together, spread across the kitchen table. Peanuts and M&M's? Salty and sweet? It was a great hands-on experience. This recipe, like so many of ours, does not require exactly all the ingredients listed. You can add more or less of each item and substitute items. This is just our general guideline to help get you started.

» 1 handful walnut halves
» 2 handfuls sunflower seeds
» 2 handfuls dry-roasted peanuts
» 1 handful dark chocolate chips or M&M's (M&M's won't melt.)
» ½ handful coconut flakes
» 4 handfuls of any of the following dried fruits: apples, bananas, pineapple, mango, cranberries, dates, prunes, apricots

In a large bowl, mix all the ingredients together with your clean hands or a large spoon. Store in snack-size zip-top bags.

We prepare our own batch of trail mix.

Lunch Day #6

Marshall: When I have brought my lunch to school, kids have made fun of me for the things I bring because it isn't cool stuff like cookies and chips. What kind of kid does that? I mean, there is no winning. Whatever I do seems to be wrong in their eyes. It's tiring.

Alex: Years ago, I worked for a temporary agency doing computer database work while attending night school. One of the places I was sent to create a database for was Nippon Credit Bank. I don't remember how long my assignment was for them, but it certainly was long enough for the Japanese senior staff, who didn't speak any English, to invite me out to lunch several times. I was amazed at the many dining customs and rituals that exist in their culture. One in particular was that they did not speak while eating. Before and after, yes, jibber-jabber galore! But during the meal, no talking because they wanted to appreciate every bite of the meal. I cannot imagine doing that at our table. Are you kidding me? It would be like a staring contest. Someone is bound to just burst out giggling. Hmmm. That could be fun!

sushi

Sushi is great because you don't really have to follow a recipe for it; you can add any ingredients you want. Anything from fish or just veggies to rice and even fruit. You will, however, need four key things: nori, the paper-thin seaweed sold in sheets; a bamboo roller; rice; and assorted items to roll inside. The nori and bamboo roller are inexpensive and can be readily found at Asian markets. When you cook the rice, you want it to be sticky. You may consider picking up some Asian sweet rice, which is actually a sticky rice, as jasmine rice will not work. I have had success by overcooking regular rice (don't use instant rice) and keeping a tight lid on it.

The ingredients should be sliced as thin as possible. This is a great job for kids. If your kids are too young to have fine knife skills, they can use a vegetable peeler on the harder vegetables to produce thin slices.

- » Carrots
- » Radishes
- » Avocados
- » Cucumbers
- » Cheese
- » Canned tuna fish
- » Red, green, or yellow peppers
- » Scallions

You may want to add a bit of flavor to the nori before you add the ingredients. Thinly spread one side of the nori with one of the following options: wasabi (which is spicy horseradish and my favorite), wasabi mayo, plum sauce (which is sweet and sour), or hoisin sauce. Just remember to start off with as little as possible, because it is easy to overpower the flavor of the vegetables.

Check the packages on your nori and bamboo rollers for directions on how to roll the sushi. I will tell you that it may take a few tries, but it's fun, it gets you busy together, and you never know: one of you little ones may have the nimble finger coordination to make a really tight roll.

Watch Marshall and Jordan build their sushi rolls.

We made sushi today and that made me think of the TV show *Iron Chef*. Well, I think I am going to ask my mom about making an *Iron Chef* night at home, where I am given some ingredients and then have to make something out of it. That would be fun. Maybe you could do it at home too!

Lunch snacks

There are some other natural and healthy snack items you can put in your lunch box that you may not have considered, such as:

» Picked okra
» Giardiniera (This is Italian pickled vegetables like you may find on a good antipasto salad. You can usually find it in regular and spicy varieties.)
» Olives
» Sweet or sour pickles
» Hearts of palm
» Pepperoncini (also available in mild and spicy versions)
» Capers
» Cocktail onions

Kids love little things that are sized right for them. Well, a bento box is a Japanese lunch box, and they usually have several little compartments. These are great fun for kids who, for one, don't like to have different foods touching each other and also love things sized right for them. Bento boxes come in many configurations and can even be found with cooling or warming sections. I suggest you visit your local Asian grocery to explore all the wonderful items there, or search for bento boxes online. They make great lunch boxes.

Like so many other food traditions, sushi began out of necessity, as a way to preserve fish for longer periods of time. Fish was often stored in rice and allowed to ferment. Then the rice was thrown away and the fish was enjoyed. Over time, the rice was eaten with the fish, and then the fish was served on top of the rice commercially. Sushi can also be considered an early version of "fast food," as stalls were created around Tokyo and "nigiri sushi" (finger sushi) was sold as a quick snack. After WWII, the sushi stalls were moved indoors for sanitary reasons.

Sashimi is high-quality raw fish served with various condiments, such as daikon radish. Sushi is basically cooked rice with a bit of vinegar in it, served with fish or other items on top or prepared into a roll with vegetables, tofu, and seafood.

What did the hungry computer eat? Chips, one byte at a time!

Lunch Day #7

Alex: Let them do it. Just let go! Don't step in and direct their imaginations. There is no lesson plan here. Let go of the desire to correct and dictate the proper method. This book and form of cooking is about creating together in the kitchen: and that creation is play. It's bonding. It's learning. It just so happens that it serves a purpose as well, and that purpose is important and has a schedule. But when you come to the kitchen with your children, think about coming to play. No one is keeping score.

cobb salad

To me, salads are yummy but don't seem to be worth the time and energy it takes to make them. Well, that was the old me, and now that Marshall is so inspired to chop and dice, a salad is a perfect lunchtime option with his help.

We've suggested a lot of possible ingredients here, but if you're missing one or two or have something else you want to add, like black beans, go for it!

» Romaine lettuce
» Boston lettuce, butter lettuce, or iceberg lettuce
» Endive (any variety)
» Bunch of watercress
» Several slices of cooked turkey bacon, crumbled
» 2 avocados, diced
» 1 whole skinless, boneless chicken breast (or chicken lunch meat), cooked and diced
» 2 tomatoes, diced
» 2 hard-boiled eggs, chopped
» 2 tablespoons fresh chives, chopped
» Few scallions, chopped
» 1 lemon

Rinse, dry, and coarsely chop the lettuce. Rinse the watercress and remove the stems, then chop. Layer all the ingredients on a large tray, decoratively arranging the food so that it looks like a rainbow. (I use my 9" x 13" glass baking dish.) Squeeze lemon juice over the salad, concentrating on the avocado in particular.

Now for the dressing. A vinaigrette with fresh blue cheese crumbled on top is typical. Use whatever healthy choice you wish. If, however, you are going to send this salad to school, you may consider putting the salad dressing on the side so the salad is not sitting around pickling in the vinaigrette until lunchtime.

Let me tell you about my favorite salad dressings. It's coconut milk and rice wine vinegar. That's it. Only two ingredients, and it is so rich and flavorful. If you do not try it here on this Cobb salad, file it away to try another time.

Watch Marshall and Alex put together their rainbow Cobb salad.

> After we boiled the eggs for the salad, my mom put aside the pot of water. I asked why, and she said she was going to use it to water plants when it cooled. She said something about recycling and not wasting. I guess we could pay more attention to that, not to waste anything. It will really help save money.

Think outside the banana box when fruit is in season. And actually, nowadays there is a lot of wonderful frozen fruit too. Cherries, plums, and apricots are good choices. And what about dried fruit? Many farmers' markets and roadside fruit stands have seasonal fruits made into preserves and marmalades. Why not send along some healthy crackers and a small Tupperware of fruit spread as a snack for school? (Don't forget the plastic spoon for spreading!)

Marshall discusses fruits he can enjoy as snacks for school.

Food Safety for Your Lunch Box

In most cases, food is stored in lunch boxes for several hours, so the lunch box needs to stay cool. Suggestions to keep your lunch box healthy include the following:

- Choose an insulated lunch box or one with a freezer pack, or include a wrapped frozen water bottle or juice box to keep the lunch box cool. By the time the bottle defrosts, it will be lunchtime.
- Follow hygienic food preparation methods. This is especially important when food will be stored in the lunch box for many hours before it's eaten.
- Prepare lunches the night before and store them in the fridge or freezer.
- Don't pack foods if they were just cooked. First cool the foods in the refrigerator overnight.
- Make sure you frequently clean and sanitize your lunch box.

Some common cutting techniques include chopping, dicing, and mincing. Chopped pieces of food are larger than diced, and diced pieces are larger than minced. Generally, chopped pieces are roughly bite-size and irregular in shape, whereas diced pieces of food are regular in shape and are roughly a quarter inch in size. Mincing is another technique that produces irregular shapes, and minced food should be smaller than one-eighth inch.

Lunch Day #8

The Freshest Salsa

I observed my big brother making this salsa about fifteen years ago, and I was appalled at his ruggedness and lack of refinement in making it. As far as I was concerned, he had glorious culinary skills, and it seemed surprising to me how he whipped this dish up. He seemed so carefree and whimsical about combining these ingredients into a wonderful sumptuous dish. So I replicated his seemingly careless (to me, that is) preparations and have made a hit salsa ever since. Thanks, big brother, for letting me figure out how to be free in something.

Ingredients are as follows, but there is one caveat: you need a good food processor for this. I have tried to make this by hand, and it really does need a food processor.

» 6 of the freshest tomatoes you can find, quartered (leave the stems on)
» Lots of whole garlic cloves, skins removed
» 1 yellow onion, quartered
» 1 bunch cilantro, rinsed (leave the stems on)
» 1 jalapeño
» Salt and pepper
» Couple squeezes lime juice
» A dash of Worcestershire sauce

Pulse all the ingredients in a food processor with the chop blade. Make sure you use the pulse setting to vary the speed so you end up with a mixture of chunky and liquidy salsa. Too much pulsing, though, and you will end up with only liquid.

This wonderfully fresh salsa can be served over eggs, vegetables, rice, noodles, steak, and chicken.

Marshall: You don't always have to be perfect in every choice you make. It's all about moderation, so keep that in mind. If you have to grab a Lunchable or something bad every once in a while, it doesn't mean you should feel like you wasted your time or that you wasted all the good choices you had made. The goal is to be the best you can be, not to be the perfect person.

Alex: I think it's natural for us humans to revert to what is comfortable, and for many of us, that is comfort foods. Chocolate. Candy bars. A biscuit and gravy. Well, now that we are concentrating on PSM, it comes to mind that this is an opportunity to actually begin defining comfort foods for our minds and our bodies. We have the choice of what we want to revert to. Is our fallback going to be the can of Pringles in the cabinet or a handful of raw almonds? The first step in defining this is to not even allow the items we don't want into the house in the first place. We are trying to change many behaviors and develop different habits, and removing temptations and difficult choices will help.

Alternate drinks at school. One day, have water; the next day, have juice; the next, milk. You will get all the nutrients you need, but you are just spreading it out instead of only having milk or only juice every day. Just take a moment to look at how much sugar is in flavored milks and juices. Yes, it may be 100 percent juice. And yes, it is real sugar. But when you look at the whole of your day, do you want that added sugar every day at lunch? And I think it's kind of unfair to pump a child full of sugar and them expect them to sit still for the next few hours in the classroom.

Tomato or Tomoto

Did you know that the United States is the second largest producer of tomatoes in the world? According to the USDA, only China produces more tomatoes in any given year. But this wide acceptance of tomatoes in the United States has not always been the case.

Tomatoes are native to South and Central America, where they were first cultivated by ancient cultures. The Spanish introduced the tomato to Europe by sending tomato seeds from the New World back to Spain, and from there, the tomato spread to the rest of Western Europe and later came to the fledgling United States.

But the fruit had a hard row to hoe after its leaves were likened to the solanales family of highly poisonous plants. This connection led to many misunderstandings and myths about the tomato. For example, in Germany, it was thought to be an ingredient in various witchcraft potions (this may be due to the hallucinogenic properties of other members of the solanales family) and shunned by the public. In the United States, tomatoes were largely thought to be dangerous as well. Several stories are reported where reputable members of society, including Thomas Jefferson and George Washington, fought to gain acceptance of the tomato as a food source. One myth talks of a noted individual who announced that he would consume a basket full of the dreaded fruit on the local courthouse steps at a specific time. A crowd of people gathered to witness the "deathly" act and were amazed when the man did not become ill or die as he ate every one of the tomatoes.

However, no matter which way you look at it, the tomato is an excellent source of nutrients for your body. It is high in vitamins A, B6, C, and K. It contains thiamin, niacin, folate, magnesium, and phosphorus. It is also low in sodium and very low in saturated fat and cholesterol. But the best thing about tomatoes is that they make a great salsa!

White Chicken Chili

This is not one of Marshall's favorite meals, but the rest of the family really loves it, and it is good for you in a lot of ways, so I wanted to include it.

» Splash olive oil
» 2 yellow onions, chopped
» Lots of garlic, minced
» 2 small cans chopped green chiles
» 2 teaspoons cumin
» Pinch oregano
» Pinch cayenne pepper
» 3 cans great northern beans
» 6 cups chicken broth
» 4 chicken breasts, cooked and diced
» 2 cups grated light Monterey Jack cheese
» Salt and pepper
» Light sour cream
» Salsa

Sauté the onions in oil over medium-high heat for about 10 minutes.

Add the garlic, chiles, cumin, oregano, and cayenne pepper, and sauté another 5 minutes.

Add the beans, broth, and chicken, and reduce the heat. Simmer for about 10 minutes.

Add the cheese and stir until the cheese melts.

Season to taste and then remove from heat. Serve in a bowl with a dollop of sour cream or some of the freshest salsa.

Lunch Day #9

Marshall: My mom told me that having too much sugar, even if it is a low-calorie sweetener, trains your brain to want more sugar.

I still want to have low-cal sweeteners, but yea, your brain cannot tell the difference between normal sugar and fake sugars, so it automatically registers the fake sugars as real sugar and makes you crave it even more to the point that you may be having diet sodas every day. Try to cut down on all the diet products. Little by little, back away from sugar in things and work to retrain your brain to stop those sugar cravings.

Alex: Do we supersize ourselves or do we portion size ourselves? That is the question! Somehow our serving size to nourish turned into as much consumption as possible for the buck. I used to purchase juice boxes for convenience, and three or four would disappear in a day. Hydration is good, but really! And I am oh, so guilty myself. I don't know how many times I justified to myself that the $5 it was going to cost to go through a drive-through was worth the amount of time and hassle it was going to take for me to make my own lunch. That thought process is coupled with the constant signage and advertisements about how much food you can get for how little money. You just cannot help yourself but to process that information and then make a decision, thinking you are getting the best value or choosing one particular restaurant just because you found a cheaper choice. It's so vicious.

Investigating Juice Boxes

Day 9
Video 1

One day we stopped at the store to pick up some juice boxes to take to school for an activity. We have learned to be quite careful: we read the ingredients and are not led by the name of the product. This is where we find it is really important to pause and take that extra moment to read ingredients. It's so easy to rush through the store and just pick up something quick. Here are some positive things to look for when selecting juices.

» If it says "100 percent juice," that is perfect. Stay away from juices that say "punch," "cocktail," or "drink."
» If the juice is cloudier, it's generally less processed and has more nutrients.

Watch Marshall compare different juice boxes at the grocery store.

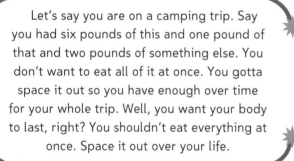
Let's say you are on a camping trip. Say you had six pounds of this and one pound of that and two pounds of something else. You don't want to eat all of it at once. You gotta space it out so you have enough over time for your whole trip. Well, you want your body to last, right? You shouldn't eat everything at once. Space it out over your life.

> I forgot this old trick somehow. I used it when my kids were young because I knew there was too much natural sugar in real juice. Now that PSM has been going on for several weeks, I just remembered it. Dilute your glass of juice with water. Just a little bit, and no one will ever notice. This cuts down on sugar and calories and increases hydration.

Beans and Wieners

It sounds old-fashioned, but what's wrong with that? This meal is easy to send to school in a thermos, and it can be used for adult lunches at work.

What you need:

- » A few natural turkey dogs, browned and cut into bite-size pieces
- » A big can of premade baked beans, like Bush's Original
- » Onion, minced (optional)

Mix the turkey dogs and baked beans and heat in a saucepan. We like to also add a bit of minced onion as well. Serve warm.

(Almost) Everything You've Always Wanted to Know about Hidden Sugars by Terri Dussault, RDH

As a dental hygienist of over twenty-five years, I have seen some damaged teeth in young people. As early as two years old, "hidden" sugars can ruin a child's dentition. Well-intentioned mothers who fill their infants' bottles with wholesome milk and allow them to snack on it for long periods of time may not realize the devastating effects lactose (milk sugar) can have on enamel. To help protect a child's first set of teeth, gently brush those first teeth the minute they are visible.

With toddlers: *watch the juice*! Remember, sugar is natural, it can be organic, and it comes in several forms—from fruit sugars to corn syrup—but the bacteria that cause dental disease *loves it all*! Ketchup is another favorite of this age group that we adults may not recognize as sugary. And not all candy treats are equal! It's the slow-melting, hard, and gooey treats that are the worst.

Now, our older children (the ones who claim they do not need any help brushing their teeth) do need help making beverage choices. Soda, energy drinks, and sports drinks can be so very harmful to teeth when consumed daily, especially when sipped over several hours. And the jury is still out on diet drinks. When it comes to tooth decay, we do agree that the flavoring acids in diet drinks cannot be good for teeth. Water is a mouth's best friend!

Isn't it interesting that the foods and drinks that are best for our teeth also happen to be good for our bodies? Did I mention digestion starts in the mouth?

Now smile and take a big bite of something good for you—from tooth to toes!

Salt pork (salted pork belly, not smoked) was used as shipboard and journey rations for hundreds of years. It can be seen in books and movies about the Civil War and the U.S. westward expansion being combined with beans in a cast-iron kettle on an open flame. It's traditional pork and beans.

Lunch Day #10

Marshall: *I'm looking forward to middle school. We got to tour it, and it was huge. I'm cool. I made some changes before fifth grade and I continue to make changes. That in itself is good, and I feel good because I am still trying to make changes. See, if I wasn't trying, I wouldn't feel good, then I would be unhappy. I'm looking at it as a fresh start. You have new people you can build reputations with. I'm a tiny bit nervous about friends, but I really am a pretty strong student, so I have that going for me.*

Alex: There was a long period of time when I couldn't even go to the bathroom without someone in the household needing me and interrupting my diligent duties. One beautiful day, I hustled everyone outside and attempted to work on a piece of furniture in the yard. Jordan, who was probably five years old, came to me and asked me for a hammer. I nervously handed it to her after I grilled her about what *not* to use it on. Then Marshall, probably three, came and asked me for a bowl. OK. I watched them scurry around the yard, picking things up, going over to the wood pile, back to the pecan tree, into the hedge. I was worried about the hammer. Mostly, I was concerned that Jordan might clunk Marshall over the head with it, worst case, or someone might get a hurt finger, best case. Time went by and I had to resist with all my ability to not ask them what they were up to. I really, really wanted to get involved. I wanted to assert my control. But I was also appreciating the time I was being allowed to work on this piece of furniture. I don't know how long went by (maybe an hour or two) while I nervously watched them out of the corner of my eye, pretending I didn't care what they were doing, until they finally came to me. Jordan handed me the bowl as they each shined from ear to ear with smiles. They had collected fallen pecans and cracked them with the hammer to remove the maggots that caused them to fall from the tree. A whole bowl full of maggots! What a prize! They were so fulfilled. Or was the prize that I didn't hover over them and tell them to be careful, that maggots are disgusting, saying, "Oh gross, don't touch that; go find something else to do"? What we are doing in the kitchen is similar. I am allowing them space to explore and discover and learn for their futures.

> There are many choices for a pudding snack to add to your lunch. One hint: if you don't have to refrigerate it, chances are there isn't much real in it. There has been a real rice pudding and tapioca product (Kozy Shack) available in the refrigerator section for many years, so I think you will be able to find it.

>> Don't deprive yourself—expand your choices!

My hardest time is when there isn't something to do or a schedule. I just immediately turn to food if there isn't something else distracting me. We figured that out and are trying things to work with that. What things have you figured out about yourself? Have you been able to figure out some ideas to help?

Leftovers are the lunch box's long-lost cousin. Usually, leftovers are lost in the haze and clutter of the forgotten kitchen. Repurposing what is in your refrigerator is a great way to keep lunches changing and save money. Silicone cupcake liners are a way to add color to your lunch box while keeping items separate and decreasing the use of zip-top baggies. If you have a leftover meat ingredient, consider sending all the sandwich elements separately so your kids can assemble the sandwiches themselves. And remember, you don't have to do this every day, but each day you or your kids pack a healthy lunch is a day they do not eat a mystery product from school.

Marshall uses leftovers to create a great lunch.

The Boxed Lunch

The vinyl or plastic lunch box that our kids carry to school today is a modern example of a truly American icon that has been around for over a hundred years. In the 1880s, as the United States industrialized, millions of workers moved from the agricultural base to the factories and mines that fed the new industrial base of the country. As they began working away from home, they needed a way to carry a hearty meal that would not only keep the food together, but protect it as well. Initially, any metal pail or box would do. Commercially made tobacco and biscuit tins provided a ready source to fulfill this need. Children also adopted these handy containers as they moved off to schools.

Over time, the commercial aspect of the lunch box was realized. In 1935, a Mickey Mouse lunch pail was introduced with the character's image emblazoned on the front. But the elaborately decorated metal box that most of us remember today really didn't get going until after World War II. In 1950, Aladdin Industries introduced a lunch box with the image of Hopalong Cassidy, a television cowboy, pasted on the side. The fantastic sales of this box led a competitor, American Thermos, to release its own cowboy lunch box featuring Roy Rogers. The lunch box boom was on. Over the course of the next 20 years, over 120 million lunch boxes were sold.

In the late 1960s, plastic began to replace metal as a cheaper manufacturing option, and in 1987, the last large-scale metal lunch box was produced. Today, most lunch boxes are made of vinyl or plastic, which fit better into a child's backpack.

Track

Helpful Hint!

One option for lightening your creamy salad dressing is to mix it or cut it with a vinaigrette. This can be a simple olive oil and balsamic vinegar mixture, or it can be a more complicated concoction, with dry mustard perhaps. Start with cutting it half and you can adjust from there, adding more creamy dressing or more vinaigrette as you like. In fact, you can have each child make their own dressing with this combination.

Your Journey!

Track Your Journey!

Ten Days of Affordable Dinners

Dinner Day #1

Marshall: You know, you guys, I'm going to tell you the truth. Without PSM, I would be on the couch right now playing my video games. They are fun, but not good for you. But really I've been inspired by my mom and everybody who has been supporting me to be more active. And I thank all of you guys for helping me get up and get more active—my mom especially!

Alex: Avoid the witching hour. Well, the kiddie witching hour. Try to eat dinner as early as you can possibly get it together. Even as early at 4:30 p.m. This allows for less stress and more time for cleanup and evening activities, such as shooting some hoops together. I find I get more cooperation if I don't let it get too late before we eat, when they start becoming little witches and warlocks with the sole intent to drive me crazy. This sounds so easy, I know. For us, it is really hard due to Jordan's soccer schedule. But we try, even if it is just a couple of nights a week.

chicken van

This meal cost us $12.03 and will feed 6 to 8 folks. One way to keep the price of meals down is to purchase a whole uncut chicken and then cut it the way you want it. In this case, we boiled it, cooled it, and then took all the meat off the bones.

- » 6 servings of cooked brown rice or quinoa (If you haven't ever tried quinoa, why not give it a shot here?)
- » 1 whole chicken, cut into pieces
- » Broccoli (This can be a bag of frozen broccoli or fresh and cut-up broccoli, uncooked.)
- » A can of low-fat cream of mushroom soup
- » A can of low-fat cream of chicken soup
- » Lots of garlic powder
- » Salt and pepper
- » Low-fat shredded Cheddar cheese
- » Slivered almonds
- » Lemon juice

Place the cooked rice into the bottom of a 9" x 13" baking dish. Layer the chicken and broccoli on top.

Mix the soups with one can of water, or leftover broth if you boiled the chicken, in a bowl. Add the spices and about two fistfuls of cheese.

Pour the soup mixture over the broccoli, chicken, and rice. Add another sprinkle of cheese plus the slivered almonds over the top. Cover with foil and bake at 350°F for about 30 minutes.

Right before you are ready to serve, take the aluminum foil off, sprinkle lemon juice over the top, and place the dish under the broiler to brown. Watch out! Those almonds will toast up quickly.

Watch Marshall go over ingredients for chicken van.

Ask your folks to load up on healthy stuff. I mean for snacks. That is the hardest time for me. It's not the actual meal but it is the snacks, and if the bad stuff isn't around, then I can pick healthy stuff that's a whole lot better for me to eat.

Green Beans

Load up on veggies. The chicken van dinner already has broccoli. But we have a lot of frozen beans from the garden, so we use them too. Boil them so they are still crisp (maybe just two minutes) and then toss a drizzle of olive oil and garlic powder over them. That's it! Keeping it simple is the best treatment for veggies.

Did you know that here in the U.S., we have approximately 230 Daylight Savings days? These are the days when the daylight is longer. If my math is correct, that is over 60 percent of the year. Time for a walk after dinner!

Green beans have worldwide appeal! Asian cooks add garlic, ginger, scallions, chili paste, and soy sauce to green beans. Greek chefs simmer green beans with onions, tomatoes, garlic, and oregano. Italian recipes include stewed tomatoes, onion, garlic, basil, and Parmesan cheese. The French love fresh young green beans and cook them gently with white wine, mushrooms, pearl onions, and garlic.

What does the buzzword "low" mean? The FDA specifies that foods labeled "low fat" must contain 3 grams of fat or fewer per serving. "Low-calorie" foods must have 40 calories or fewer, and "low-sodium" products must have 140 milligrams or fewer per serving. The FDA does not define "low sugar," so that term can be applied to anything.

Dinner Day #2

Marshall: This process takes amazing amounts of courage. Just like soldiers in war, eating healthy and exercising is like a war. You need courage! I know most kids go trick-or-treating on Halloween. Does it take courage to walk up to that door, knock on it, and say "trick or treat" to a complete stranger? So don't think of these new healthy changes as something that scary. Think of it as you're gonna get a reward—you're gonna feel better and be healthier, so that's sweet. That's your treat.

Alex: I really couldn't be any prouder of Marshall. I am so excited for his future. I have no idea if he will be a lawyer, fisherman, scientist, chef, or politician. He may end up being a professional gamer. I really couldn't tell you, except that I am confident in the knowledge that he will be colorful and dynamic in whatever he chooses to do. I feel very privileged and grateful to be his mother. He has his moments, don't get me wrong, but he overwhelmingly adds richness and exuberance to my life. I am prepared and excited to see his future unfold.

Nachos in a skillet

I think nachos seem more American than Mexican. I'm not taking away from Señor Nacho (Ignacio Anaya, the inventor of nachos, nicknamed Nacho Anaya) and his creative efforts to prepare whatever he had in the kitchen for his guests. It's just that every bar and restaurant in the United States seems to have a nacho variation. Ours here is yet another version, and the goal is to avoid eating too many tortilla chips. This entire skillet meal cost us about $11, and it provides plenty of leftovers for lunch the next day.

- » About 1 pound lean ground beef or our previously mentioned half-and-half mixture of lean ground beef and/or lean ground turkey or chicken.
- » 1 onion, diced
- » Lots of garlic, chopped
- » Taco seasoning or just salt and pepper
- » Can of low-fat refried beans
- » Tomatoes, diced
- » 1 bunch of cilantro, rinsed and chopped
- » Scallions, chopped
- » Black olives, chopped or whole
- » Spoonfuls of wholesome jarred salsa or some of the freshest homemade salsa (see Lunch Day 8)
- » Avocado, diced
- » Lime juice
- » Hot sauce
- » Shredded low-fat Cheddar, mozzarella, or pepper jack cheese (whatever you have)
- » A few spoonfuls of light sour cream

Brown the meat with the onion and spices in a deep dish that can go in the oven (a cast-iron skillet is perfect).

After the meat is cooked through, layer whichever of the remaining ingredients you desire on top. (If you're using refried beans, it's okay if it's a bit lumpy when you spread it around. If you choose lime juice or hot sauce, sprinkle the liquid around lightly on top of your meat mixture. If you choose cheese, make sure to lightly scatter it on top.)

Put the whole pan underneath the broiler for about 6 minutes, keeping a close eye on it. If you want to get fancy, you can stick tortilla chips randomly one-quarter of the way into the dip, leaving the rest exposed to get gently toasted by the broiler. But you must watch this very closely. **Watch Marshall give directions on making Nachos in a Skillet.**

This process is like fighting a war. You cannot go into a war afraid! You wanna make a change. Stand up and take charge! Nobody is in charge but YOU!

What can you do with all those tomato stems and cilantro and scallion ends? Well, we take ours out to feed to the chickens. But if you don't have chickens, you can compost them. If you don't have or want a big composting routine, purchase a countertop jar that you can put all your food scraps in. After a week or two, when it gets full, you can dump it on your plants or herbs outside. The mixture has already started breaking down, and it will quickly share its nutrients with your plants or herbs.

Watch Marshall tend to the family chickens.

Lazy Sorbet Dessert

Take a can of frozen 100 percent fruit juice concentrate and prepare it according to the directions on the can. Pour into a deep glass dish and put in the freezer. You must stir it every once in a while as it freezes to keep it from settling. Once frozen, use a sturdy spoon (not your finest silver one) to scrape pieces and curls off the top of the dish. Place the sorbet into your ice cream dishes and enjoy. It's light, simple, refreshing, and *real*.

Marshall enjoys his homemade sorbet.

You have probably noticed that we use the herb cilantro quite often. I think it is one of our favorites. It has a very fresh and light taste to it without overpowering other flavors. This herb is used in Asian, Latin American, Caribbean, and U.S. cooking. It can be found fresh year-round in the produce section of the grocery. Be careful not to mistake it for parsley; they are often put next to each other and it's easy to pick up the unintended one. It can be quite sandy, so it must be washed thoroughly and kept in the refrigerator. It is also easy to grow on your own.

Courage: the attitude of facing and dealing with anything recognized as dangerous, difficult, or painful, instead of withdrawing from it; the quality of being fearless or brave; valor.

Dinner Day #3

Marshall: Sometimes when I'm bored, I find I get hungry for no reason. In order to stop boredom while watching TV, try getting some play modeling clay so that you can sit there and play with it in your hands. Sometimes they come with a tool that you can use to make a face or a figure, or you could use a toothpick. Then you can mix it all up and start all over so that you are not wanting to do something with your hands by eating. You could do the same thing with Legos 'cause you can build and rebuild. Customize them in many different ways. You could try writing, especially during the commercials. Write about what you're watching or how you feel. The point is that you keep yourself occupied and not thinking about food.

Alex: I have mentioned some unintended benefits happening with PSM, and I have discovered another: my kids have strengthened listening skills and a greater tendency to follow directions. These are learned skills, and not only will they assist kids in life and in school, but they should continue to ease your job at home. I know, I know; it is taking a lot of patience on your part. I also know you know in your heart that the payoff is good.

Fish Tacos

I've never really cared for fish tacos at restaurants, and it is mainly because I don't care for the coleslaw that is usually served with them. Something about the mayo or Miracle Whip used turns me off. So I figured out a way to make them with shredded cabbage, onion, and cilantro and no mayo, and they were fabulous. Give it a try!

» Bit of butter
» Several tilapia fillets (or you can use another white fish)
» Fresh lemon juice
» Salt and pepper
» 1 or 2 squeezes of fresh lime juice
» Green or red cabbage, shredded

» Red onion, chopped
» Cilantro, chopped
» 1 can black beans, drained
» Corn tortillas
» Low-fat shredded cheese
» Hot sauce (optional)

Heat the butter in a skillet and add the fish. Season with the lemon juice and salt and pepper. Cook over medium-high heat for about 5 minutes on each side, or until the fillets are cooked through and a little crispy. Put aside but keep warm.

Mix together the lime juice, cabbage, onion, and cilantro, and chill while you finish preparing the rest of the recipe.

Heat the black beans in the microwave until they are quite warm. When the beans are heated through, use the microwave to warm up the corn tortillas.

Now put a couple of pieces of fish in the warm tortilla, cover with the warm black beans, add a sprinkle of cheese, and then top with the chilled slaw mixture. You may consider adding a dash of hot sauce if you like. *¡Buen provecho!*

Grilled Corn

This is heavenly, and you can be very creative with it. Each child can make his or her own special corn. Corn is usually in season all summer long, and when it is, it can often be found in the husk. That is how you want it for this recipe.

Grab as many good-looking ears as you want, and carefully pull back the husk without breaking it or removing it. Gently remove the threads along the ear and any remaining inside the husk. Gently replace most of the husk around the corn, leaving a place to put in some goodies. Yup, you're going to add your favorite things to the corn, inside the husk, and then roast it on the grill or in the oven.

If you add any fatty element, like butter, you should put the corn onto a piece of aluminum foil so it doesn't scorch. On that note, some of the husks may catch on fire. That's OK; just move them over on the grill and blow the flame out. When the corn is done, your husk will be black all over, and that's just fine. It should take about 20 minutes on a hot grill or about 30 minutes in the oven at 350°F. Now consider these combinations to stuff and season them with:

- » Salt, lime juice, and diced onion
- » Salt, cayenne pepper, and onion powder
- » Salt, lime juice, and a bit of butter
- » Salt, pepper, and Parmesan cheese
- » Zesty Italian salad dressing
- » Thinly sliced mushrooms

 Marshall preps grilled corn.

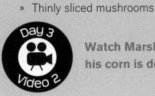 Watch Marshall determine when his corn is done.

Throughout Europe, "corn" has always been the generic name for any of the cereal grains. Europeans call what we refer to as corn "maize," a derivative of the early Native American word *mahiz*. In fact, before settlers came to the New World, Europeans had never seen this food—called "Indian corn" by colonists. What a wonderfully versatile and useful gift the Native Americans gave the world! Everything on the corn plant can be used: the husks for tamales, the silk for medicinal tea, the kernels for food, and the stalks for fodder.

Is it dangerous to swim on a full stomach? Yes, it's better to swim in water.

Dinner Day #4

Who Flong Bean

We used to call my sister, Pilar, "teeny eeny weeny beanie." When she made this wonderful meal, we also coined a clever name for it: "Who Flong Bean." Not really sure why, so let's move on. This meal cost about $10 to make and easily served 4.

» 6 lean pork chops (boneless is best)
» Pepper
» Garlic powder
» Seasoned salt
» 4 broccoli stalks, chopped
» 1 medium onion, diced
» 2½ cups cooked brown rice
» 3 tablespoons chicken bouillon or the equivalent in cubes

Place the pork chops in a skillet and generously season both sides with the pepper, garlic powder, and seasoned salt, as this will add a lot of flavor throughout the dish. Cook over medium heat, covered, for approximated 6 minutes on each side. Then remove the lid and cook on medium high until the chops are browned and cooked thoroughly. Cool and cut into bite-size pieces. Set aside.

In the same pan, add about 1 inch of water and begin to simmer, scraping all the pork chop bits and crusted seasoning off the bottom of the pan. Add the broccoli, onion, and pork chops. Mix together, cover, and cook over medium heat for just about 5 to 10 minutes, or until the broccoli is tender.

In another saucepan, cook the brown rice with bouillon in water. Add the brown rice to the pork chop mixture. Cover and heat on low until warm, just a few minutes. You want your broccoli to have a slight crunch. Serve.

Marshall: We haven't talked too much about portion sizes. A portion size is the amount of food you are supposed to have. It's usually not in our mind to think about our portion size; we just eat until we are full, right? Here are a few tips I've learned. Let's say you are having a serving of corn. Well, it should be about the size of your fist. A piece of steak or meat should be the size of the palm of your hand. Nobody ever thinks about the portion size. They order the thirteen-ounce sirloin and think that's right. A cup of food would be like the size of a baseball, and if you are having oils or something that's an ounce, it would look like a cube from a pair of dice. Just remember to eat small amounts and don't fill your full meter all the way up.

Wisdom from Aunt Pilar (aka Aunt Pepper): A mind-set is needed to stay away from fast food. I have found that when I frequent fast-food places I seem to want it more often. When I practice no fast food, I can stay on my diet longer. Fast food gives me a lazy mind-set and then it takes time and strength to get back on the right track and reset my mind-set to a healthier one. I personally seem to go through phases like that. Being good for a while and then not being so good for a while. I can't quite figure it out, that is to say if I am in a healthy mind-set phase, why can I not stay there? I wonder if other people feel the same way or have the same patterns. I am hopeful for Marshall to stay on track with his current positive mind-set so that he doesn't go through the same swings I do as an adult.

I have looked at some packages, and I think they try to hide the labels. Or sometimes you just don't think about looking at the serving size. I like a certain bottled green tea, and I just figured it was one serving. But actually, it is two and a half servings. Now I look closer and I immediately look at the servings so I understand. Then the other day we saw something at the store called "Apple Straws." It had pictures of apples on the cover and it was in bright green letters. We looked at the ingredients and it wasn't that bad. EXCEPT! There were no apples in it, just apple flavoring.

Chili

This is a down and dirty chili my big brother used to make for himself.

Take a can or two of regular premade chili. Just make sure to read the ingredients and make sure everything in it is real. It can be turkey chili or meatless chili.

Then add a can of stewed tomatoes. Again, check the ingredients: sometimes they sneak stuff into stewed tomatoes, especially if it is flavored, like Italian style. You can add half a can of diced chiles to it; they don't have to be spicy hot.

Heat all the ingredients to a slow boil, and voilà: you have a quick and easy spruced-up version of chili.

Most canned chili is like eating wallpaper paste, so this is a way to lighten it up a bit, and it is very inexpensive.

This Little Piggy Went to Market

The tried-but-true saying that everything but the pig's squeal can be used is accurate indeed. Though pigs are bred primarily for their meat (commonly referred to as pork) and fat, the trimmings and lesser cuts (feet, jowl, tail, etc.) are used for sausage, the bristles for brushes, the hair for furniture, and the skin for leather.

The majority of pork in the marketplace today is cured—like bacon and ham—while the remainder is termed "fresh." Slaughterhouses can (but usually don't) request and pay for their pork to be graded by the U.S. Department of Agriculture (USDA). The grades, from highest to lowest quality, are USDA 1, 2, 3, 4, and utility, and each designation is based on the proportion of lean meat to fat. Whether graded or not, all pork used for interstate commerce is subjected to state or federal inspection for wholesomeness, ensuring that the slaughter and processing of the animal was done under sanitary conditions.

Today's pork is leaner (about one-third fewer calories) and higher in protein than the pork that was consumed just ten years ago. Thanks to improved feeding techniques, trichinosis in pork is now also rarely an issue. Normal precautions should still be taken, however, such as washing anything (hands, knives, cutting boards, etc.) that comes in contact with raw pork and never tasting uncooked pork. Cooking it to an internal temperature of 137°F will kill any trichinae. However, allowing for a safety margin for thermometer inaccuracy, most experts recommend an internal temperature of 150° to 165°F, which will still produce a juicy, tender result.

Dinner Day #5

Marshall: You gotta try new things! You cannot just be set in your ways, or you will never have new experiences. Sometimes even your tastes change. I used to not like white chicken chili, but my mom made it the other night again and this time I liked it. I don't know how that happens but if it does, just go with it! I know I used to say I didn't like things just because I hadn't heard about it before. But then I tried it and was surprised. That's why these days I like Korean food, sushi, and all kinds of stuff.

Alex: This is such a wonderfully wholesome process. There is something comforting about getting back to basics. It feels safe. It feels right. And it feels solid. Don't be surprised if your child and family don't quite feel as if they are in the same place as you are. It is scarier for them because they are following the new path of consistency in healthy behaviors you are carving out. And even if they don't enjoy a few of the recipes you make together, they will enjoy the process with you. And they may even feel fulfilled by the process more than the actual consumption of the food itself.

Curry Lentil Soup

You can make this recipe with or without ham. If you chose to include ham, you might try cooking a whole ham, eat it for one meal, and then use the leftovers and the bone to make a stock for this lentil soup, leaving all the meat that has fallen off the bone. You can also add prepackaged diced ham pieces. Below is the recipe without ham, and it cost us only $8. If you add the ham, which we strongly recommend, it will cost a few more dollars. But if you purchase a whole ham or a portion to cook for another meal and just use the leftovers for this one, then you are getting a double bang for your buck.

- » 2 packages dry lentils, separated
- » 8 cups stock (If you don't use ham to make a ham stock, then use chicken stock.)
- » Several celery stalks, chopped
- » Several large carrots, cut into bite-size pieces
- » 1 large onion, chopped
- » Lots of fresh garlic, chopped
- » Several dashes of curry powder
- » Salt and pepper to taste
- » 1 bay leaf
- » Fresh cilantro, chopped

Rinse the lentils well in a colander. Add 1½ packages of dry lentils to the stock and simmer for about 30 minutes, stirring frequently.

Meanwhile, sauté the celery, carrots, onion, and garlic until the onion just becomes transparent. Add the sauté mix to the stock. Add the curry powder, salt and pepper, and bay leaf to your pot and simmer for another 15 minutes.

Next add the remaining ½ package of lentils to the pot and simmer for another 15 minutes.

Taste and adjust the seasonings. (I usually add more curry powder here.) Continue to simmer until you are happy with the seasoning and texture. Cool a bit, serve, and garnish with a pinch of fresh cilantro.

Watch Marshall discover what happens to all the fat after a ham is cooked and refrigerated.

One thing that I want to tell you is that pets are great friends and they are great exercise partners. They can be super playful, and you take them (dogs) out in the yard and play with them. You can spend time with them and train them. You could even train them for certain exercises and jogging. Dogs make excellent jogging partners like what I call my dog...Mr. Jog Dog.

That gets you exercise and helps you out. Always play with your pets even if they won't jog with you. They love to spend time with you.

Marshall gets some exercise with his favorite pets.

Day 5 Video 2

Nutella Tapioca Pudding

Nutella is a hazelnut cocoa spread found near the peanut butter section in the store. Many folks spread it on a piece of toast, but here we are combining it with some tapioca pudding. Tapioca is derived from the cassava plant whose root is also used for many things, including dessert.

Make the tapioca according to the box directions, but use low-fat milk and add a little less sugar than the box suggests. When it is almost finished cooking, add in a bit of Nutella and stir well. Don't worry if all of it doesn't seem to melt. Little warm bites of it in the tapioca are delicious. Let the mixture cool for 20 minutes, and then serve. You can also put this in sundae glasses, cover with plastic wrap, and keep it for a snack in the refrigerator.

Garlic

Garlic has been used as a natural remedy for thousands of years. From the ancient Egyptians to the modern Americans, garlic has been a staple not only in cooking, but also in myths.

To the Egyptians, garlic was a treatment for stomach disorders and fertility problems. In Southeast Asia, hanging a string of garlic and chilies in a doorway is thought to protect against the entry of evil spirits. Likewise in Europe, hanging a string or bunch of garlic in a child's room is thought to do the same.

Today, raw garlic is used in some cases to treat the hardening of the arteries, high blood pressure, and high cholesterol. It also has a certain level of bacterial fighting capability and was used to treat the spread of infection during World Wars I and II.

A more questionable use of garlic has been its use in the treatment of parasites within the human body, usually in the digestive system. Some people believe that garlic has the ability to either drive the parasites out or even protect against the parasite in the first place. While modern medical science may support the basic antiseptic properties of garlic, there is little to support anything beyond that.

However, there has been proof through the ages that garlic can protect against at least one large and serious parasite: vampires!

Dinner Day #6

Marshall: In my opinion, dinner is the hardest time for portion sizes. You wanna know why? It's because what I think is, "Oh, my gosh, it's the last meal of the day and I have three more hours to go before bed so I better eat a lot and stock up." So like bears do for hibernation, we stock up, but the problem is that we are not bears. We don't need that much to get through the night. We sleep; we don't burn off all that we ate. We don't need to eat so much at night or such heavy stuff. I mean I really love mashed potatoes. They are making me hungry right now just thinking about them. But do we need to have them every night? Or cheesy stuff every night? Fatty meats? Gravies? I have heard that eating that heavy is the "American way." The American way is apparently to get fat on your bed watching TV all day long. Not good. I will be honest and say that this is always hard for me. I have not mastered it yet. I have to keep thinking about food and fuel.

Pork Tenderloin Barbeque

This unfortunately is not an affordable dinner that you can pick up at any time, but if you keep your eyes open, pork tenderloins do go on sale quite often. And I would even suggest picking up a couple extra tenderloins when they are on sale and keeping them frozen. I don't care to purchase the ones that are preseasoned, as I like to do that part on my own. Here is how:

» 1½ cups balsamic vinegar
» Lots of chopped garlic
» Several sprigs of rosemary
» Salt and pepper
» Couple pinches of dry powdered mustard
» Pork tenderloin

Place the balsamic vinegar, garlic, rosemary, salt and pepper, and dry mustard in a large zip-top bag and add your pork tenderloin. Marinate for as long as you can; overnight is wonderful.

Now you can grill this tenderloin, or you can put it in a covered roast pan (with an inch of water in the pan) and cook it slowly in the oven at 350°F for about 1 hour, or until cooked through.

Alex: I understand that when dating, one is trying to explore the interests of the other. I also understand that eating out can feel like an indulgence or a special treat: either to try something new or to have a break in the routine. And I can understand a husband and wife literally trying to get some quiet time at a noisy restaurant. But why take your kids? I'm not talking about the special occasion or where you are trying to teach them manners. But some folks seem to take their kids out weekly or multiple times a week. I am just curious about how this is fulfilling. Is the cost to entertainment ratio equal? My family has a tendency to eat very fast so we can spend a lot of money in a short period of time at a restaurant. It just seems to me that several hours together in the home kitchen is a bigger bang for the buck...and you have leftovers.

>> This is a multifunctional idea. If you find yourself using or particularly liking a group of herbs and spices, why not premake your own mixture or shaker of it? You'll have it ready

anytime you need it. Try having your child mix all the ingredients you like into a bowl and then use a funnel to put them into a shaker. Depending on your child's age, you can make this super easy or make it a mathematical formula to reinforce what he or she is learning in school. Yet another benefit of this idea is that you will no longer have to have so many spice tins or jars taking up space in your cabinet. You'll just have one with everything you like in it.

> We have discovered that our afternoon snack after school needs to be bigger so that when dinnertime comes around, I'm not starving and don't wind up overeating. I think it's also a good strategy to drink lots of water after school. I don't get to drink that much water at school and that's a long time to go without.

Mac 'n' Cheese

We tried to make a healthy, whole-wheat version of mac 'n' cheese, and, well, let's just say we need to keep working on it. But Marshall's friend Adam suggested that we choose Annie's brand mac 'n' cheese over the regular boxed kind. I looked at the ingredients, and we think it's OK to keep in the cabinet. One thing that I noted about the ingredients is that it said "organic wheat shell pasta." That is not whole-wheat pasta. It may have been made with wheat flour, but carefully recognize that that is not whole-wheat flour. Also, portion control comes into play. Each one of us could eat the whole box, but one box is two and a half servings, and should be noted.

BBQ

Some people say that the technique of BBQ, or slow cooking meat to make it tender, originated in the American West during the last part of the eighteenth century. In an effort to feed cowboys without using the best, most expensive cuts of meat, the lower quality cuts were served, such as brisket. These cuts were less than tender and flavorful, so slow cooking the meat for an extended period tenderized it. Others claim that the practice of slow roasting meat evolved in the Southern United States in the pre–Civil War era.

No matter where it started, adding seasonings and spices to flavor the meat and then slow cooking it eventually evolved into BBQ and led to the creation of BBQ sauce.

Different areas of the country have different styles of BBQ. For example, the Southeastern United States is known for sauces made with a vinegar base, while the Midwest uses a tomato base. There is even a recipe from Hawaii that uses pineapple juice as a base!

Dinner Day #7

sticks and all that stuff, but somehow it's affecting my body more. Yes, it frustrates me. It makes me feel like I want to take the easy way out. I would like for it to be easy, like it seems it is for other people. But there are so many things in life you have to deal with. This may be my struggle, but other things come easy for me. Those things that are easy for me may be difficult for other people. So I guess it's all fair and that's why I try not to compare myself to other people.

Alex: Way back when, little boys plowed and picked the fields alongside their fathers and little girls canned, cooked, and took care of animals. During the Great Depression, children helped by cleaning the house, sewing, cleaning vegetables, and perhaps trying to sell things for spare change for their family. In the '50s, even as distractions like TV and radio grew in prominence, kids took out the trash, mowed the postage-stamp-sized yard, and washed dishes.

Today...how often do we ask our children to help around the house? Maybe we ask them to take out the trash once in a while. Marshall's job is to unload the dishwasher each day and scoop the cat box. Together, this may take ten minutes. That used to be his only contribution, but now he helps in the kitchen. Assigning chores may be old-fashioned, I suppose, but it feels good and helps our family. Who says old-fashioned is out of style?

Beer Can Chicken

The kids find this recipe funny because I don't think they believe me that all the alcohol cooks out of the chicken, and they think they are secretly getting intoxicated. And it's fun to stuff something as large as a can into a bird and precariously set it upon a grill or in the oven. You know...the small joys of adulthood and childhood! Truthfully, the alcohol does burn out and the remaining liquids steam the chicken from the inside. You could use soda or a can of iced tea instead of the beer.

- » 1 whole chicken
- » Lots of garlic, freshly minced (or lots of garlic powder)
- » Salt and pepper
- » Dry mustard
- » Rosemary or thyme
- » 1 can of beer (or soda or iced tea)

Rub the chicken with the garlic, salt and pepper, dry mustard, and rosemary or thyme.

Insert the open can of beer (or whatever you choose) into the chicken. It helps to have one person hold the bird up and another insert the can so you don't spill the liquid when trying to do it yourself.

If you are going to cook the chicken in the oven, place the bird in a deep roasting dish and set it standing up so that the can is upright and not spilling. Bake at 425°F for about 45 minutes to an hour, basting occasionally. I like to pull on a drumstick, and if it pulls off easily, I know it's done.

If you are going to do this on your grill, wrap the tips of the drumsticks with foil so they don't brown too fast and carefully place the chicken on the grill, using the wings to support its upright position. Cook over medium-high heat for about 45 minutes, watching carefully that some parts aren't cooking too fast.

Watch Marshall prep beer can chicken.

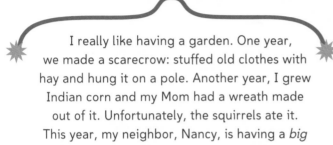

I really like having a garden. One year, we made a scarecrow: stuffed old clothes with hay and hung it on a pole. Another year, I grew Indian corn and my Mom had a wreath made out of it. Unfortunately, the squirrels ate it. This year, my neighbor, Nancy, is having a *big* garden and letting me have my own row in it. Even if you live in the city, you still can grow some things. Basil and rosemary are herbs we grow really easily. We grow grapes too, as well as blueberries, but the birds always eat them first. You should give gardening a try! Don't go crazy, just start with one or two things you want to try.

Mashed Rutabaga

I didn't grow up eating a lot of root vegetables, and I believe my mother introduced mashed rutabagas to me in adulthood for Thanksgiving. Surprisingly, the kids like it for its slightly tangy taste.

Wash, peel, and quarter a couple of rutabagas. Boil them until they're soft, just as you would do with mashed potatoes. Add a smidge of butter, light sour cream, a splash of skim milk, and salt and pepper, and mash, again just like you do with mashed potatoes. Use more light sour cream in lieu of butter to achieve the consistency you want. I usually add more pepper than I do with mashed potatoes, and I love to have slivered almonds on top.

Glycemic Index

The glycemic index is an indicator of the ability of different types of carbohydrate-containing foods to raise blood glucose (sugar) levels within two hours. Foods containing carbohydrates that break down most quickly during digestion have the highest glycemic index value.

Root vegetables have always been a key nutritional staple as they are the storage vessel, the holding tank, for all the fuel for growing the plant and they store longer than other types of vegetables. Rutabagas are a cross between a turnip and a wild cabbage.

Do chickens think rubber humans are funny?

Dinner Day #8

Alex: In U.S. culture, the Thanksgiving holiday is an annual reminder of the bounty that we receive. It takes place during the traditional harvesttime, the fall. Many families come together and prepare a large, traditional meal. Special attention is paid to family recipes, and often, this is the only time of the year that certain foods are served. But why is this concept of celebrating the harvest limited to once a year or special occasions? Shouldn't we give our food this attention throughout the year? We should really try looking at the foods that we eat on a daily basis and honoring them. We should focus on selection and preparation to ensure that our daily foods are balanced and nutritious, and therefore special.

Leek & Squash Soup

- » 1 bunch leeks, washed and chopped
- » 2 tablespoons butter
- » 2 acorn squash, halved lengthwise and seeds removed
- » Couple pinches of thyme (Fresh is best, but dried is OK.)
- » 5 cups chicken broth
- » Lots of fresh crushed or powdered garlic
- » Couple pinches of salt
- » Several pinches of pepper

In heavy saucepan melt butter and add leeks and thyme. Stirring occasionally, cook covered on low/medium heat for about 40 minutes until soft and browned.

Heat oven to 350°F. Place acorn squash on baking sheet cut side down and roast for about 40 minutes. When done, cool so that you can handle them.

Stir stock into leeks and, using a spoon, scrape out the inside of the squash and also add to the leeks. Add salt, pepper, and garlic. Simmer for about 15 minutes. In a blender or food processor, puree the soup in batches until smooth. Pour the soup back into the pan and cook for another few minutes; then it's ready to serve.

Meanwhile you can prepare some garnishes like fresh cilantro, chives, scallions, homemade croutons, crispy bacon, fresh tomatoes, and even a bit of light sour cream. Whatever you wish and have on hand.

Artichokes

I grew up in California, and while researching for this book, I discovered that globe artichokes are predominantly grown there. Who knew I was so spoiled with good food growing up? I recall eating them quite often, and now I eat them so infrequently because I only have access to tiny specimens compared to what I recall growing up with. Anyway, they are super easy and super delicious, and they take patience to eat.

When purchasing artichokes, make sure they are firm. They shouldn't look too beat-up but don't worry about the first couple of outer leaves. Boil a large pot of water and add a dash of salt and a few whole peppercorns if you have any. When the water is rapidly boiling, add the artichokes and cover to keep the water at a constant boil. They will take about 25 minutes to cook. The leaves will gently relax and spread as they cook, and the way you tell they are done is to remove a leaf as close to the center as you can grab (without burning yourself); if it slips off easily, it is done. Let cool.

Now to eat! Peel off a leaf and dip the tip closest to the core of the artichoke in a low-fat rémoulade; light, zesty Italian dressing; or balsamic vinegar. Then use your upper or lower teeth to scrape the meat off without biting through the leaf. Work your way all the way down the artichoke until the leaves are too small to grasp.

Next, grasp the remaining clump of leaves and tear them away from the round heart. Use a teaspoon to remove any remaining tiny leaves (and the hairs) from the bowl of the heart, and enjoy the artichoke heart. You have worked hard to get to this glorious spot.

See Marshall and Jordan pair a whole artichoke with leftovers to create a balanced and filling meal.

Also, Marshall teaches you how he eats artichokes in these videos.

> OK, so now you have done and tried some new things in the kitchen! Why don't you plan a meal all by yourself? Any day can be Mother's Day. Why don't you surprise your mom?

More Kitchen Lingo

Simmer means to cook a liquid until bubbles just start to break the surface.

Boil means to heat until bubbles rapidly and regularly break the surface of your liquid.

Scalding is half of the steps of blanching. When you **blanch**, you submerse something into boiling water and then into ice-cold water. To scald is to just quickly submerge in boiling water and then set aside. You might do this to remove the skin from a tomato.

Steam means to cook your food with steam, so it must be held over boiling water in some sort of rack or basket in your pot.

Dinner Day #9

Marshall: We don't do it too much, but I like to use the tools in the kitchen. I don't mean the microwave, but the mixer or food processor and stuff. Like when we make salsa, we use the food processor. We use the blender for smoothies, although that one makes more noise. It's fun. It's like using power tools in the kitchen. I even know that we have an electric carving knife. But I have never used it. Maybe one day for Thanksgiving!

Popeye Soup

» 1 tablespoon butter
» 1 yellow onion, chopped
» 1 turnip, peeled and chopped (This thickens the soup and adds a unique "bite" to it.)
» Lots of chopped garlic
» 3 bags of spinach or 3 fresh, big bunches of spinach, washed and dried well
» 6 cups chicken stock
» Salt and pepper

Melt the butter in the bottom of a large stockpot and sauté the onion, turnip, and garlic for about 10 minutes.

Add the spinach leaves and cover, allowing the vegetables to cook for about 20 minutes and stirring occasionally.

Add the stock and simmer another 10 minutes.

Now comes the tricky part. You need to run the mixture through a blender, so you will need another pot. The way I do it—and yes, it makes a bit of a mess—is to ladle the soup into the blender, blend well, and then poor the pureed mixture into the new pot. Repeat until all the soup is done.

Return the soup to the heat and simmer for about 10 more minutes, adding salt and pepper to taste.

Alex: When I was a kid, I was taught manners, like serving to the right of a seated person and clearing to the left. As an antiques dealer, I have learned that the Victorians created a utensil for every single purpose, though today we find some of them unnecessary. My children, on their own, are now learning about presentation of food and how to be a host or hostess. Well, they might be getting a little bit of it from me, but they are taking time and care when assembling a plate. It is now important to them to take pride in their dishes and finish all the way through until it's eaten. I don't mean "finish" the food, rather finish the whole process of creating a meal. They plan, they prepare, they present, and they enjoy. When they serve, they serve everyone, and they think ahead to any condiments that may be wanted. It's another unintended, yet positive, benefit of Portion Size Me. Now if I can just get them to clean up after themselves...

> Have I told you that this fun? I mean, who wouldn't want to learn how to cook some things. Your mom can't take care of you forever, you know.

»» Marshall's comment on power tools in the kitchen brings up an idea. Why not have a tool themed cooking day where you make recipes using particular appliances and teach your kids how to use them safely? My kids don't even know how to use a toaster oven. I better get on that one.

Go Ahead, Play with Your Food

While we largely regard food as sustenance on a daily basis, have you ever considered food as art? Many natural food items have been used to decorate for many years. For example, the Native Americans used various berries to dye their clothing and decorate their bodies for ceremonies. In the Shaker religion of the American East, blueberries were used to produce the traditional blue paint that became a staple color for their furniture and houses. Likewise, milk paint, which is a mixture of milk, lime, and pigment, has been used for thousands of years to decorate.

But how about more modern examples? Do you and your family use food to decorate during holidays? When the main table is set for the holiday dinner, the food is presented in an appealing fashion, often on the best dishes available (you know, the fine china that only sees the light of day once a year). The dishes are arranged and coordinated with the centerpiece to become a true work of art for everyone to enjoy before digging in. At our house, we have fruits and nuts in the table centerpiece during Thanksgiving and Christmas. Some people use gingerbread cut into shapes like stars and men to decorate their Christmas trees. We build a gingerbread house, decorate it with bright candies, and display it through the holiday.

In a more common form, the birthday cake is an expression of art. If you watch the latest craze of cooking shows, you see some really amazing examples of cakes that are presented not as food, but as art. And what kid doesn't love a cake frosted in bright colors and adorned with the latest popular cartoon character, set ablaze with colored candles and surrounded by wrapped gifts?

All of these examples showcase food in a place of significance, not as food but as a decorative form of expression. This is just one more reason to think about food in our life.

Homemade Croutons

For this recipe, I use bread that is on its way out. This can be leftover hot dog buns, sandwich bread, or pita pockets. Cut the bread into chunks and toss it in a bowl with salt, pepper, garlic powder, and a pinch of red pepper. If you like herbs, feel free to toss some dried ones into the bowl too. Heat 2 tablespoons of butter in a large skillet, and when it's hot but not burning, add the seasoned bread chunks. Keep tossing and turning gently in the skillet until the bread begins to dry out and crisp up. Make them as crispy as you want. If the pan is getting too dry before the bread crisps up, add small amounts of olive oil to keep the croutons from burning. Serve with the Popeye soup.

Certain dishes, like soups, require a thickening agent due to the high moisture content in the product. Flour, cornstarch, egg yolks, yogurt and vegetables, such as turnips and potatoes, can also be used to thicken and add additional flavor to your dish.

Dinner Day #10

Marshall: It was very scary for me to have to rely on myself for these big changes. Even though my family has been with me, there are still some things I have to face on my own. I was tired of how I was feeling. The changes have kinda been scary. It's like a big blue abyss. It's the unknown. You don't know what's down there until you get down there. I realized I had to do it. And it's fine. It's not scary anymore. Once you try, you realize it's like a roller coaster. You have ups and down but it's a fun ride.

Beef stroganoff

» 1 pound or so of lean sirloin steak or top loin (Whatever is on sale and is lean!)
» 2 packages fresh, sliced mushrooms, separated
» 1 onion, chopped
» Lots of garlic
» Salt and pepper, to taste
» Splash of white wine (optional)
» Small container light sour cream
» 1 package whole-wheat egg noodles

Cut the beef into thin strips. In a large skillet, brown the beef with half the mushrooms and the onion, garlic, and salt and pepper. Once the beef is browned, drain any fatty liquids and add the remaining mushrooms. Take the skillet off the heat.

Add the wine, if you so choose, and fold in the sour cream. If you don't add wine, you may need another liquid to make the sour cream creamier. You can add a tiny bit of water or beef broth. You have to judge based on how the dish is coming together for you. Bring the mixture to a simmer and let it cook while you prepare the noodles in a separate pot.

Once the noodles are cooked through, lightly toss them in olive oil, and then spoon the stroganoff over the noodles and serve. This meal will have a lot of leftovers.

Alex: More and more benefits keep cropping up of getting the kids more involved in the processes, planning and preparation of meals. During these ten days of affordable dinners, they have learned so much about the cost of food, prioritizing, and making decisions to meet our financial goals. The shopping experience itself has, I hope, benefitted Jordan the most, as she seems to be the one with the least amount of respect for currency. Marshall has always been quite frugal with his personal birthday and holiday monies and has no difficulty saving his money for things he wants. He also did not have any problem giving things up at the grocery store to stay on target. Think about it: when do we as parents ever really spend time educating our children about real-world dollars and cents? Sure, we may talk about bills and such, but that is a foreign concept to most children. No wonder so many kids get to college and then rack up large credit card bills.

What is the thing you have never had but wanted? Not a toy. Something inside you, like courage. Today, you can feel worthy and reach out and grab for it. Just go for it! My mom has been saying, "You can't change without making a change." Do you get it?

> When shopping for beef, the darker the meat is, the better it is for you. It means less marbling of fat within the meat.

Roasted Green Beans

This is so simple and extremely delicious. I would try it even if your kids have declared that they don't like green beans. Just gently toss some fresh green beans in olive oil and a dash of salt (kosher or sea salt is awesome) and spread out in a heavy-duty baking dish. Roast in the oven at 450°F for about 10 minutes. Turn the beans over and roast again for another 10 minutes. That's it.

What Do the Labels Mean?

Here from the USDA's Food Safety and Inspection Service (FSIS) is a glossary of meat and poultry labeling terms. FSIS is the agency responsible for ensuring truthfulness and accuracy in the labeling of meat and poultry products. Knowing the meaning of labeling terms can make purchasing meat and poultry products less confusing.

The term "certified" (e.g., "certified angus beef") implies that the USDA's Food Safety and Inspection Service and the Agriculture Marketing Service have officially evaluated a meat product for class, grade, or other quality characteristics. When used under other circumstances, the term must be closely associated with the name of the organization responsible for the certification process (e.g., "XYZ Company's certified beef").

The phrase "no hormones administered" may be approved for use on the label of beef products if the producer provides sufficient documentation to the agency showing that no hormones have been used in raising the animals.

Curdling, which is when milk proteins coagulate and lump together, can occur in any dairy product. This causes separation of the curds (the protein lumps) from the remaining liquid. Several factors can cause curdling, including the addition of acids, tannins, or bacteria or using a high cooking temperature.

You can avoid curdling in a number of ways: Avoid using acids, such as lemons, or tannins, such as coffee. Heat cream sauces slowly and avoid bringing them to a boil. Add a pinch or two of flour to cream sauces, as flour protects against curdling. If your sauce does curdle, whisk it vigorously and remove it from the heat while continuing to whisk.

Track

Helpful Hint!

Sometimes my sister and I drink hot tea. This also helps with that urge to eat, and it's really warming on cold days.

Your Journey!

Fun Fact!
The fish symbolizes many things. For example, in Christianity, the fish symbolizes the abundance of faith. In China, the fish is symbolic of unity and fidelity. And if your birthday is in the winter and your zodiac sign is Pisces, your symbol is two fish.

Track

Helpful Hint!

Here is a fun thing to do to think about portion sizes. Go to a dollar store and pick up some half dozen muffin pans. They can be disposable aluminum or hard aluminum or even those somewhat flexible, silicone ovenproof muffin pans. Then use them as old-fashioned TV dinner trays. Use each muffin hole for a serving of something and even put a small cup with your drink in one of them. Good, plain fun!

Your Journey!

Track

Helpful Hint!

We have previously suggested not keeping foods you don't want in your body in your pantry because the temptation is too great. However, what if your family is accustomed to having dessert? It may be too difficult to remove that treat completely from your routine. Consider having a dessert night once a week or even twice a week if need be. Setting dessert nights ensures your family doesn't overindulge in after-dinner treats and also gives you something to look forward to. You could even alternate times when different family members get to pick what dessert is.

Your Journey!

Curry Powder:

Widely used in Indian cooking, curry powder is actually a pulverized blend of up to twenty spices, herbs, and seeds. Among those most commonly used are cardamom, chiles, cinnamon, cloves, coriander, cumin, fennel seed, fenugreek, mace, nutmeg, red and black pepper, poppy and sesame seeds, saffron, tamarind, and turmeric. (The latter is what gives curried dishes their characteristic yellow color.) Since curry powder quickly loses its pungency, it should be stored, airtight, no longer than two months.

Track

Your Journey!

Helpful Hint!

Make a color theme for a meal. Challenge yourself and your kids to make a whole meal out of green things, or purple things, or red things. It will really tax your eyeballs at the store and may even help you to try something new (like white eggplant or white asparagus to go with your white chicken chili).

closing

Good-bye from Alex

What you have found in these pages is the unflinching truth of one modern family living in a world dictated by their schedules and technology, two precious children, pets, school, soccer, friends, jobs, hobbies, extended family members, and more. As we showed you, we have pulled together as a family to rediscover and relearn what the household kitchen is for and how it united us as a family in the most wholesome and nutritional sense. We hope we have inspired your sense of adventure.

As a result of this sixty-one day journey, Marshall has removed himself from the obese category. I have dropped pounds too. Jordan no longer has stomachaches from plumbing issues. I feel confident that we have learned tremendous amounts about ourselves, about each other, and about our futures. We have physical energy and an energy in spirit—perhaps that's called excitement or stamina. Dan will return soon, and we are all looking forward to being a family unit again and sharing our newfound tools.

I am so very grateful for the support of dear family and friends who helped organize and contribute to Marshall and me putting our videos, thoughts, and ideas down on paper to share with you. The written contributions from Dan, Pilar, Terri, Leslie, Dr. Bryan, and Jenks pale in comparison to their actual emotional support to me and Marshall. Although their written contributions are wonderful additions to this book, please know that they spent additional efforts in supportive roles and for that I am very thankful. Terri worked hard to help me translate the confusion between my brain and the emotions in my soul into words that could be understood. Dan's research skills were invaluable.

I should say too that Marshall and Jordan have really put up with a lot that I would consider outside the normal childhood experience. They have been subjected to some unique stressors and exciting situations: twice interviewed live on CNN; a trip to NYC for an appearance on *The Nate Berkus Show* where they surprised Marshall with an introduction to Chef Jamie Oliver; and multiple local appearances and interviews. They are resilient young people, and I hope they are enjoying their childhoods for all the robust experiences they encounter. I love them dearly and I am exceptionally proud of them.

Good-bye from Marshall

Thank you for reading this book. These last few months has been hard but I've pulled through it all. This is going to sound sappy, but the truth is I could not have done this without you! I've wanted to quit multiple times but I thought if I quit, what would the viewers and readers think? You would be disappointed, so I said OK, I need to keep going, so I did. One thing I have learned is to trust myself and I want you to trust in yourself too. Maybe I mean confidence instead of trust. But I mean that you don't have to be scared to make some of your own decisions and now I know, and you now know, how to make some of the decisions.

So I want to thank you very much for reading this. You helped me so much and I hope I have helped you too. So please keep in touch with us at www.portionsize.me or on YouTube.

And, see you in my next book!

About the Authors

Marshall, an avid reader, enjoys military history, video games, and building things.

First-time author Alexandra Reid is the mother of two, Jordan and Marshall, and the wife of Lt. Colonel Daniel Reid. A former advertising executive, she now dubs herself the jack of all trades and master of none, spending most of her time taking care of house and home (Rancho Reid), kids, an antiques business, and hobbies, all with a multitude of military deployments. When asked what her biggest attribute is, her response is: "I'm a very good cheerleader for my family, friends, and causes." After cheerleading the development of this book with her family, they have moved on to their next creation, FreeSeedsForSchools.com, an Internet-based game to educate youth about health and nutrition while earning seeds for schools who want to start gardens.

Recipe Index

Snacks

Dinners

Sides or Appetizers

Beverages

Desserts